The Health Evolution

Why Understanding Evolution is the Key to Vibrant Health

The
HEALTH
EVOLUTION

Why Understanding Evolution is the Key to Vibrant Health

Dr. Stephen Hussey

To my parents

For my father, who guided me toward an inquisitive nature and fascination with science, and my mother, who inspired in me a desire to do good in the world and taught me to have an optimistic outlook.

Contents

Prologue

"The test of a first-rate intelligence is the ability to hold two opposed ideas in the mind at the same time and still retain the ability to function."

– F. Scott Fitzgerald

If there was ever a poster child for inflammatory illness, it was me. By the age of twelve I had experienced asthma, allergies, chronic hives, irritable bowel syndrome, and the autoimmune disease, type 1 diabetes. These inflammatory conditions were terrible to go through, especially at such a young age. However, I find myself unable to completely resent them. Those early experiences in poor health fueled my desire to look deeper into why they happened to me, especially when the explanation my medical training offered wasn't quite satisfactory.

Aside from my collection of illnesses, I had a pretty usual upbringing in my small western North Carolina town. I had a good group of friends, a love for sports, and a healthy desire for snow days. I got my teenage heart broken, attended church with the family on Sundays, and had many adventures in the wilderness courtesy of my outdoorsy father. When my senior year came, the obvious choice was to go to college like all my friends.

Because K-12 had come easy to me, I got a wake-up call the first semester of my freshman year. After nearly failing two of my classes, I realized I had no idea how to study and had no choice but to quickly learn. Ironically, one of the courses I nearly failed that first semester was Ecology and Evolution—a topic you will hear a lot about in the coming pages. Please don't reference my freshman year transcript when deciding if I am qualified to write this book!

Looking back, I feel that I was largely unprepared for college because in school I had never been encouraged to pursue my own curiosities. It felt like school was about only learning what was required to pass standardized tests. I was soon to find out that most of my college professors were counting on me to engage in complex thought processes. Unfortunately, my early schooling had not been designed to teach me to think. College required more than trying to memorize and regurgitate.

I spent so much time mastering the art of passing a college class that it took me until my senior year to fully understand that the world is intriguing and that I could follow my own interests to learn about it. By then I had switched majors twice. It wasn't until I developed an interest in health that I felt connected to my pre-med curriculum. I found that health could be related to any class, no matter the topic. With this I started to find success in academics. However, as graduation approached, I became way more concerned about how my girlfriend and I were going to stay together.

In my attempts to stay close to her I ended up applying to a chiropractic school near where she was going to school in Oregon. My parents had taken me to chiropractors when I was younger, and medical professional school had a lot to do with health, so I figured it was a good move. So, in 2009 I moved to the West Coast for two things—chiropractic school and a girl. The two of us, her allergy-inducing cats, and my brother crammed into the cabin of a moving truck and headed west. That relationship ended after a few months but my new surroundings expanded how I saw the world, and learning so extensively about the body further intensified my passion for health. I still couldn't quite pinpoint why I was passionate about it. I just liked learning medicine and keeping myself healthy. I discovered that it was very easy to control type 1 diabetes when I paid attention to my lifestyle, and I found it curious that this approach to managing diabetes had never been mentioned by any of the endocrinologists I had seen over the previous fifteen years.

Even as I was learning all the anatomy, physiology, bio-chemistry, radiology, orthopedics, diagnosis, and clinical skills that are required to be a doctor, I found myself wondering if this was all there was to know about health. I felt that there had to be more than what was being taught but I didn't know the right questions to ask. One night, I struggled to convey to my roommate some of my thoughts on how huge facets of health and medicine were missing from medical school curriculum, but when she asked me to elaborate I couldn't provide an answer.

It took until my third year of clinical practice to truly find out what interested me most about health. I guess I don't like to rush things. By then I had backpacked through Central America and practiced chiropractic and functional medicine in Europe for two years. I learned that no amount of travel would ever satisfy me because it fueled a newfound passion. I am extremely interested in humans—more specifically; why society and the natural world we call home is the way it is today and how it differs for people in different cultures and geographic locations. How did the things that *now are reality* come to be, and how has this impacted health? Anthropology and health are, in fact, very interconnected—who knew? Just as I couldn't quite engage in pre-med until I became interested in health, I couldn't understand my passion for health until I applied it to human societies, past and present. Now I can weave the threads together; throughout all of my schooling and research, way back to that freshman ecology and evolution class, I have become acutely aware of the decline of health in Westernized cultures, and I wanted to learn how to best combat that decline. Being born into one of these chronic disease-stricken societies, I have personally felt the effects.

Health is much more complicated than diet, exercise, and stress. Through examining the varieties of human experience, including my own, I have come to realize that an individual's state of health is a direct result of their environment and overall human experience. Drastic events and environmental changes have caused many of our contemporary health struggles. Knowing how human life fits within the context of evolution is also vital for understanding how to combat disease. These realizations have altered my life, influenced my approach to guiding patients back to health in my clinical practice, and taught me that we humans have much more control over our health than I was taught in medical school. It is now clear to me that in the places where Western medicine fails to shed light on the reasons for our chronic disease epidemic, ecological and evolutionary ideas light a clear path.

All of the topics in this book—such as chronic disease, major flaws in our healthcare system, evolution, and socioeconomic inequality—have affected my life and led me to the conclusions herein. Many doctors, including me, are tired of practicing in our broken healthcare system. We are discovering new ways of offering care that seeks to help patients achieve well-being instead of pursuing solely the absence of symptoms and the profit of the conventional medical system. As much as this new approach to health makes sense to many healthcare practitioners, its true potential will not be reached until it is understood by everyone in the general public. The better part of a century of misinformation about health has created a healthcare system based on false information and has left the general public lacking the knowledge and tools necessary to lead a life that creates optimal health. This book attempts to bridge that gap.

A Note on Methodology

You will find that this book is not like most health promotion books; it could be described as a health philosophy book. Most health promotion books use an arsenal of research to make their point. By citing research, one can "prove" to anyone that, for example, changing their diet will result in stable blood sugar better than taking a pill,[1] and that exercise is better for depression than any anti-depressant drug will ever be.[2] However, I feel that proving something to you with quoted research and statistics is, in a way, superficial, because there is also research out there that says that medications are better for those conditions. Therefore, while I will cite research, I will attempt to keep the research and statistics talk to a minimum. If I did tell you to look at research to form your health opinions, I would also have to tell you to investigate who funded that research and what their agenda might be before you decided to trust the results. There is a huge conflict of interest in the world of health and medical research.

Further, research only provides various facts and figures resulting from experiments—it doesn't give instructions on what to do with those facts and figures, and it definitely doesn't show you how those facts and figures relate to the grand scheme of things. To make things sink in a little deeper, a more philosophical assessment is needed. A philosophical assessment of why our health is declining, and why lifestyle change, as opposed to Western medicine, is the best answer. In the coming pages we will see how this deeper understanding is essential, not just for the sake of each individual person's health, but for the survival of a species living within a rapidly changing global environment.

In a way, I don't want anyone to believe a word I say in this book without scrutinizing it for the truth. The information I present has been earned through my experience, training, and education. But we each have to make our own hard-earned journey to the truth. If something I say leaves you doubtful, contradicts what you think to be true, or stirs any kind of emotion in you, I encourage you to do your own health research or health experiments and prove to yourself that the response you had was valid or not. My goal is not to prove one way of thinking or another but to share with the world the thought process that has given me the personal answers I was looking for and has allowed me to better the world by helping others reach their health goals.

A Note on Evolution

There is a lot of evolution talk in this book, and my conclusions rely on a fundamental acceptance of evolution. Since I realize that not everyone agrees with this particular theory I have a favor to ask. If you do not accept the theory of evolution, please do not dismiss the overall message of the book or the parts of the book that can help people achieve health and create a better world. I hope that those who do accept the theory of evolution will also not condescend to those who don't. It is my belief that if we respect each other, we will find ways to constructively discuss across beliefs.

Reflect back on what F. Scott Fitzgerald is quoted as saying at the start of this prologue. Friedrich Nietzsche once had similar thoughts. He said, "The wisest man would be the one richest in contradictions, who has, as it were, antennae for all types of men—as well as his great moments of grand harmony—a rare accident even in us!" Based on the words of these two men, I hope that those who are confronted with ideas in this book that contradict their beliefs see that they do not have to change their beliefs to benefit from the information; they merely have to see potential benefit in understanding different interpretations of the world.

The Chapters Ahead

In the coming chapters I will present why we need to think differently about our approach to health. Part One sheds light on the epidemic of chronic health issues we find in the world today, especially in the West. We will explore the responses from Western medicine and why these responses are flawed and dangerous. In Part Two, we will dive into evolution for an explanation as to why we are experiencing this epidemic. We will review some evolutionary principles, take a look at the history of human evolution, use these lenses to explore answers to the health decline, and then look at the consequences of staying on the path we are now on. With this foundation, we will then see how evolution not only gives us an explanation but also a solution to our health issues. In Part Three, we will explore strategies that can help the individual achieve greater health while having a positive impact on the world, and show why it's not as hard as everyone thinks. Finally, I will present you with the most convincing proof I have come across that this is the most effective way to achieve health.

I wrote this book for two reasons. First, I want to help others achieve an optimal state of health. And second, I want to bring awareness to the positive affect that achieving optimal health can have on society. We all deserve optimal health, and we can each be our best self when our biology is functioning at its optimum.

Part One:
The State of our health

Chapter 1: An Extended Stay in the Hospital

I have always had a good memory; I even have a memory from when I was still in my crib. My dad can't believe it, but I vividly remember him coming in to comfort me back to sleep because I had woken up crying. It's interesting how different memories stick in our heads more than others. One memory has become more and more important as my life has gone on, especially because of the route my life has taken.

*****

I was sitting in an exam room at Dr. Riley's office. My mother was sitting by the door and I was turned a little away from her, facing my pediatrician. I was nine years old. I liked this doctor's office because it didn't smell as sterile as others I had been to. I had been to Dr. Riley's office many times—not only for the usual checkups but also for the many ailments I had as a child—allergies, hives, asthma, and intestinal discomfort. This visit felt different though.

Recently I had been feeling lethargic, and my muscles felt kind of crampy all the time. I distinctly remember being in school, especially in the computer lab, and feeling "funny." I would have to get up to go to the bathroom more than my peers, and the look

Miss Greene would give me made me think she thought I was up to something. After these symptoms persisted, my mother decided to take me to Dr. Riley.

I remember looking up at him in the exam room and noting that he had a different tone to his voice. Instead of his usual carefree and playful approach, he was much more serious. He was staying positive, but there was obviously something going on that he knew a steroid or anti-inflammatory medication—my usually treatment—would not cover up. Though he was trying to use nine-year-old words, I didn't really grasp what he was saying. To this day I don't remember the ins-and-outs of what he said, but his tone made a lasting impression on me.

He was directing what he said more toward Mom and my mind started to wander—I starting thinking about what my friends at school would be doing right now—when I heard him say that I would need to be admitted to the hospital by the afternoon. I had never been to the hospital before and my initial reaction was joy—my nine-year-old self immediately thought this meant I didn't have to go to school today. When I turned to ask my mom if this was true, I noticed that she was crying.

Mom and I stayed in the hospital for the next week or so as they taught us how to control type 1 diabetes and monitored me while I took my first doses of insulin. This week had many ups and downs. On the up side, my nurse, Ken, was super cool and taught me my first ever magic trick, which I still use to impress kids today. I had visits from friends and family members who brought me nice things like cards and toys. My brother thought I was going to die because the disease is called die-abetes, which offered some comedic relief after we assured him it wasn't that serious. On the down side, I caught the virus that was floating around the pediatric floor of the hospital and had a pretty rough couple of days. I remember wondering what a bowel movement was after being told that I would need to tally them on a white board in my room. I also had to prick my finger to check my blood sugar five times a day. They drew blood numerous times for tests, and I had to get an IV when I caught the virus because I was dehydrated and couldn't keep fluids down. I remember telling my mom that I felt like the pincushion in her sewing kit at home.

When I finally got home I had to quickly adapt to some new things. Finger pricks and insulin shots were now a daily part of my life. These few weeks were a defining time in my life—not only because of the day-to-day changes of controlling diabetes, but because in the long run it changed the course of my life. Looking back, I see that having diabetes has always made me wonder *why*. As a nine-year-old, I wondered "Why me?" That evolved into "Why do I care?" when I was a teenager. Finally, in higher education, I began to ask, "Why did my body react this way?"

My early childhood experience introduced me to our modern world's epidemic of chronic diseases—diseases that Western medicine deems incurable and that must be managed throughout the duration of a person's life. As a kid with diabetes I was given lots of diabetes education and I went to a few diabetes camps. I always felt like everyone was trying to show me and the other diabetic kids that we weren't different and that this was a normal thing that happens to some kids. I have learned that having chronic diseases at such a young age has sadly become much more common in the Western world, but it is not normal. Nor is it normal for adults to suffer from chronic disease, especially at the rates that they do today.

Chapter 2: Twenty-First Century Illusions of Health

"It is more important to know what kind of person has the disease, than what disease the person has."

-William Osler

Up until about eighty years ago, when antibiotics were invented, the threat of infectious disease was an ever-present danger facing our society. The world had already seen extensive death at the hands of infectious diseases like "the Black Plague" in the mid-1300s and thousands of years of smallpox outbreaks. Infectious diseases have been the nemesis of humankind since the first groups of humans formed farming communities ten to twelve thousand years ago. Living in such close proximity to each other and to livestock exposed us to dangers that we could not see with the naked eye. Close confinement made waste management and hygiene—issues we humans never really had to pay attention to when living wild in small groups—a real concern. These issues remained a problem until the very recent past.

After discovering that microbes passed between living beings caused infectious disease and devastating outbreaks, human ingenuity harnessed the power of nature to produce a weapon that greatly reduced the amount of life lost to this kind of disease. The study of a naturally occurring mold lead to the discovery of penicillin, the first antibiotic. This string of discoveries transformed human society and revolutionized medical treatment, public health, and personal hygiene. As a result, in developed countries, the average life expectancy rose from the mid-forties at the beginning of the 20th century to the mid-seventies today. [1]

Many people credit most of this rise in life expectancy to the advancements in modern medicine. However, I think that the measures taken in public health and personal hygiene have had just as much, if not more, to do with this rise. As will be reiterated in the book, it is far better to avoid getting a disease than to try to counteract one once it has taken hold of us. While antibiotics gave us a tool to combat an infection, the knowledge of where they come from and how to avoid them was just as important in our quest to conquer them.

As much as this medical revolution was able to save lives, it exposed an issue that had been hiding from us. Infectious disease was causing the death of so many people at what we would consider a young age that it was obscuring the effects caused by ten thousand years of radical changes in lifestyle and personal environment. To put it another way, if you have a house that has a mold issue, termite infestation, and a poorly built foundation, and it suddenly burns down, you are not going to see the long-term effects of the mold, termites, and foundation and probably will never even know they were a problem. It was impossible to notice that lifestyle and environmental changes were spawning an epidemic of chronic decreased health when there was a much more effective killer on the loose. Infectious disease was beating chronic disease to the punch, so much so that even doctors and medical researchers didn't notice.

Although infectious disease is not the threat it once was, we are now confronted with an epidemic that has been silently growing right under our noses. The result of our medical system being so distracted by the battle against infectious disease is that we now have an underdeveloped healthcare system that is poorly equipped to handle an epidemic of *chronic disease*. Our medical system has limited knowledge as to the cause, development, and treatment of these diseases.

Chronic disease acts very differently from infectious disease. It does not kill us as fast as infectious disease; it kills us much more slowly and causes a lower quality of life for a much longer time. One recent response to chronic disease that has come from outside of Western medicine is termed functional medicine. In functional medicine, chronic diseases are known to have four characteristics:

1. They do not heal by themselves, like the common cold does;
2. they get worse over time, especially since modern healthcare has ineffective ways to treat them;
3. they typically don't have a single cause but multiple causes;
4. and they tend to display complex sets of symptoms that can send a clinician down an unclear path of diagnosis.

You can see how different this is from the usual scenario of, "You have an infection; take this medicine to kill it."

Because antibiotics were so successful at combating infectious disease, medicine has tried to duplicate this approach with whatever ailment it has encountered. For any number of diseases or symptoms your doctor will prescribe a pill to cure your ill. But for a century this approach has proven wildly unsuccessful. It is estimated that 40% of all Americans—133 million people—are affected by chronic disease.[2] The medical community is very quick to take credit for our increased average life expectancy over the last century; however, while they have put out the fires of infectious disease, something insidious has been taking a hold of our health and, recently, a decline in average life expectancy has been predicted.[3] This decline is due to the increasing prevalence of chronic disease, the appearance of chronic disease at earlier and earlier ages, and our poorly equipped medical system.

In the forward of *The Disease Delusion* by Dr. Jeffrey Bland, Dr. Mark Hyman states:

> Chronic diseases now affect one in two Americans and accounts for 80 percent of our healthcare costs. Yet despite a host of new drugs and procedures, the incidence of chronic disease continues to rise, not only in the United States but around the globe as developing countries adopt the worst of our food and culture.

The diseases Dr. Hyman speaks of include asthma, Alzheimer's, allergies, autism, ALS (Lou Gehrig's Disease), acid reflux, Addison's Disease, ADD/ADHD, anemia, angina, anxiety disorder, arthritis, atherosclerosis, and autoimmune disease—and those are just the A's I can think of off the top of my head. Chronic disease is taking over our society, and I fear that one day soon we are going to end up like the people in the movie WALL-E, too unhealthy to do anything but ride around in mobile chairs, with screens in front of our faces, eating our "food" from a cup.

Health is declining on a global scale; however, it is much worse in the United States. The United States ranks worse in health than other Westernized wealthy countries such as Australia, Canada, France, Germany, the Netherlands, New Zealand, Norway, Sweden, Switzerland, and the United Kingdom.[4] The consequences of us continuing down this road are many, and it is important to first recognize that there is a problem. After all, admitting we have a progressively worsening epidemic is the first step.

Being as immersed in the health world as I am, I see the effects of our health epidemic on a daily basis, but I remember a time when I was oblivious to just how bad it is. I want you to do a tiny experiment this week. From the time you wake up until the time you go to bed each day, I want you to count how many times you hear someone complain of a health issue. Count how many times you hear someone say anything along the lines of, "I have a headache," "I'm tired," "so-and-so is in the hospital," or "I just can't shake this cold." Take notice of how many people you see that look like they are struggling with their health. How many people do you see who are overweight, have trouble walking, or just look like every ordinary day is a hard for them? Once you start paying attention, you'll soon realize how prevalent these situations are. You will also start to realize that it is not just certain groups of people that are impacted, but that every age, race, and gender is being afflicted by poor health.

Likely, you could even just look at your own family to see how widespread chronic disease is. Take mine for example. One of my grandfathers suffered with cancer and cardiovascular disease, another suffered from a form of Alzheimer's, and one of my grandmothers struggled with COPD and diabetes for years before her death. All of them died relatively early in life. Not to mention the numerous aunts, uncles, cousins, and extended family members who have everything from chronic pain to heart disease to Meniere's disease. Hell, even I have type 1 diabetes. Ah, the follies of an inflamed youth! My point is that as normal as it may seem for us to be surrounded by these diseases, it is not normal. When you think about it, the whole thing is insane. If an ancient society had experienced the same drastic rise in symptoms over this relatively short period of time, they would probably think their gods had turned on them and would be performing every ritual in their repertoire to please them. We, as a society, seem to be content with the dismal results we get from going to our primary care physicians and accepting that our poor health is just the way things are.

Even people that modern medicine would call generally healthy have days that go something like this:

> After dragging themselves out of bed, it takes at least half an hour to finally feel awake. They may or may not eat breakfast, but they cannot function without their morning caffeine, which they continue to consume even after lunch because coffee just switches to soda or energy drinks. If they did eat something for breakfast, it was something convenient like cereal, fast food, or a doughnut. Halfway into their morning they have a headache, can't focus, and seem irritable. The only thing that seems to help is a sweet snack from the vending machine. They manage to get a little something done before lunch, and even get a little boost from lunch, only to crash at about 3 or 4 o'clock. They are getting another headache late in the workday. This time it feels like the light in the office is causing it. After an unmotivated and unproductive day at work they know they should hit the gym because they are starting to put on weight, but they are so exhausted they can't even fathom it. It is again pushed off until "tomorrow." Once they get home they order out because they are too tired to cook and then spend the rest of the evening catching up on social media or the latest TV shows. They decide to go to sleep early tonight because they feel like they are getting a cold only to find that when they get in bed, it feels like it

takes them forever to fall asleep—they are just wired for some reason. They finally fall asleep and tomorrow they get to wake up and do it all again.

Headaches, fatigue, lack of motivation, extra weight, and insomnia are just some examples of the many things that plague "generally healthy" people every single day. If these people went to their doctor and got a full workup, it is very likely that everything would come back normal and they would get a clean bill of health. We will discuss more about why doctors come up with a "generally healthy" label for these people in the next chapter, but in brief, it is because doctors are trained only to identify and treat disease. Therefore, if you don't have a full-blown, diagnosable disease, then many doctors have nothing to offer you. You are left with the label of "healthy," despite struggling in the day-after-day cycle described above. You will come to understand the causes of this struggle in the coming pages.

Needless to say, the typical day of a "healthy" person outlined above does not sound healthy, or enjoyable. If a life filled with those ailments sounds bad, imagine what condition you would have to be in for our medical system to officially say that you have something wrong with you. In order to actually treat a patient, doctors have to have enough positive symptoms or test results to make a diagnosis and provide a treatment, but just because someone may not have positive results leading to a diagnosis doesn't mean they are healthy. The truth is, our "generally healthy" population is just around the corner from a full-blown ICD 10 approved medical diagnosis. In the words of Jeffery Bland, the founder of The Institute for Functional Medicine:

Disease has its start as a functional impairment (a dysfunction) that, left untreated, becomes a diagnosable disease that later can become the cause of death. Each disease has a past, a present, and a future tied to the progressive loss of function and vitality.

With few other tools at their disposal, doctors in Western countries have been giving out diagnoses in shocking quantities. After all, when all you have is a hammer, everything looks like a nail. I know this analogy is true because as a kid, when I used to "help" my dad on construction projects, he would hand me the hammer to keep me occupied only to take it back ten seconds later because I would be hitting anything in sight—the table, the dog, my sister.

When someone does end up with a medically approved diagnosis they may enter our healthcare system, only to never get out. Someone getting Western medical treatment may experience a cascade of diagnosis that go something like this:

They first go to their doctor for a regular wellness visit, which they expect to go without incident, as it usually does. However, this time their lab tests show an increase in the thickness of their blood. The doctor doesn't speak of why this is, he just tells them that this puts them at risk for a heart attack and decides to place them on a blood thinner. They listen to their doctor and take the blood thinner because the abnormal blood test scares them a little. Unfortunately, unbeknownst to the doctor or patient, this blood thinner depletes their body of vitamin K. Six months later, the doctor notices that the patient has decreased bone density, probably because of the decrease in vitamin K, and recommends that the patient goes on either hormone replacement therapy or an osteoporosis medication. The doctor does not realize that both of these options can result in excessive loss of vitally important minerals. After six months of losing minerals due to this new drug, along with a diet high in refined sugar that the doctor did not think to address, the patient develops elevated cholesterol. Upon seeing this, the doctor recommends a statin drug to lower cholesterol. These statin drugs reduce cholesterol in the blood by halting cell division and tricking the body into storing cholesterol in cells. This causes problems in places like the brain and muscle tissue, because these are places that depend on high rates of cell division, and the patient ends up with memory problems and muscle pain. Also, since cholesterol is tied up in cells, the body cannot use it to make sex hormones and the patient eventually ends up with sexual dysfunction. The doctor will likely prescribe drugs for each one of these issues.

You can see how this can keep building and building. There are many different variations of this, and it all could have been avoided if the doctor had known that the patient could have achieved the desired effect of thinner blood by making diet and lifestyle changes.

Major chronic diseases like heart disease, cancer, COPD, diabetes, and neurologic conditions have been on the rise for the good part of the last century and they are still rising. New "diseases" like chronic fatigue syndrome and fibromyalgia are starting to pop up as well. Our health has gotten so bad that medical associations are being forced to make up new diseases to match new patterns of symptoms they are seeing. If you have any connection to the health community, this rise of disease and symptoms is not news. The statistics of the rise in disease quoted above are telling, but observing the health epidemic happening in your local community is eye opening. It would be easy to read the statistics and say "wow," then keep reading and forget about them. If you open your eyes and really see how widespread these health problems are, then it's more likely to stick with you. Perhaps you will see that those people you see who are suffering aren't much different from you. You may then understand that even if you don't suffer from a chronic disease right now, it could happen to you just as it did to them.

We will talk about genetics much more in later chapters, but briefly, I want to squash the idea that genetics cause disease. Our rise in chronic disease and general lack of health has only appeared in the second half of the 20th century. If we combine this realization with the fact that our genes have not changed at all during this time, then it does not makes sense to explain our increased incidence of chronic disease by blaming it on our genes. We now know that our genes are very much influenced by our environment. Therefore, it is much more sensible to question how the major changes in our environment and way of life have affected our health over the years.

Further, through the work of the human genome project it was discovered that a large proportion (I have read anywhere from 96-98%) of our genes are identical to that of our closest relatives, the chimpanzees. This raises more curious questions about our lack of health, as chimps do not experience cancer, or heart disease, or autism. It was thought that examining those genes that we have that are different from chimps would shed light on why we experience disease but they don't. While studying that 2-4% difference in genes has explained many of the differences between us and chimps, such as our advanced cognitive skills and ability to speak, nothing has been found that explains why we get complex chronic diseases and they do not.

Does our epidemic of disease mean that humans are really that poorly evolved compared to chimps? Why did chronic disease in humans rise so drastically only recently when we have been around for at least 200,000 years without it? Why for the first time in recorded history is a child born today not expected to live longer than their parents did? Did our genes just give up on us?

One silver lining is that chronic disease does not kill us quickly. This gives us time to counteract or even reverse its process. But due to this characteristic of chronic diseases, they cause many years of suffering leading up to death; some even have these diseases for more than half their lives. These people require many years of care, and this care costs us trillions of dollars per year in our country alone. It is also costing people large amounts of wages from missing work. Paradoxically, despite spending more money to treat these diseases than any other country in the world, they are still on the rise. Curiously, the people who benefit the most from this spending are not the patients but the pillars that make up our medical industrial complex: the pharmaceutical companies, the insurance companies, and the healthcare providers. The healthcare industry is quick to promise an easy fix, but following the money reveals why, despite spending more on healthcare than any other country, the United States still has the unhealthiest population in the world. Sick is not the default state of the human species and we should not accept it as normal.

Chapter 3: Diabetes Strikes Again

I remember waking up on the cold, unforgiving hospital room floor. Eleven years had passed since I was diagnosed with diabetes. They had not all been easy years. I continued to struggle with inflammatory conditions such as chronic hives, asthma, and irritable bowel syndrome; I had converted from insulin injections to using an insulin pump, and like most teenagers who can't foresee the long-term consequences of their actions, I had not taken care of myself to the best of my ability and had become angry with my parents when they tried to help me.

Despite all that, I had managed to avoid any repeat visits to the hospital until now. By now I was in college and the day prior to waking up on the hospital floor I had gotten a call from my mother saying that my older brother was having symptoms. He had to urinate multiple times during the night and was so thirsty he was drinking water by the gallon. Given my experience 11 years before, we all knew what this meant; he was likely also type 1 diabetic.

My father and I dropped everything and drove down to Charlotte, where my brother was in school and had been admitted to the hospital. His tiny hospital room didn't have much space, and since he was in the bed and my dad was in the chair, I was left to make do on the floor. Awaking and coming to my senses the next morning, I noticed the familiar sterile smells and medical equipment sounds of a hospital that had gone unnoticed in the whirlwind of the night before.

As nurses and doctors came in and out of the room, many of them commented on how unusual it was for a 22-year-old to be newly diagnosed with type 1 (juvenile) diabetes. At the time, I was fairly certain that there was nothing I could have done to prevent this from happening to my brother. It would be years before I learned how it could have been prevented.

There was nothing much to do but sit with my brother as he learned to manage his new disease, so my dad and I decided to pay my old pediatric diabetes specialist a visit to see if he had any recommendations for an endocrinologist that my brother could see. I had really liked my pediatric doctor and was sad to have to move on from him once I turned 18. He went to great lengths to help his patients and did everything he could to help children feel special. He was conveniently located in Charlotte, more or less across the street from the hospital. When we arrived he graciously came out and spoke with us, even though we dropped in unexpectedly, and gave us the name of a colleague he knew and trusted.

It's strange now to remember how I felt back then. I had complete faith in the Western medical system to help me and my brother manage this autoimmune condition. I remember thinking that they knew everything—that this was just something that happened to us, and they were the heroes that could get us through. My, how things have changed. It's not that I am not thankful for everything every employee I encountered in the Western medicine system has done for me, it's just that I can now see how broken that system is, how their training falls very short when it comes to achieving optimal health, and how the system has failed an uncountable number of people.

Chapter 4: Medical Incorporated

"The sense of futility experienced by many healthcare providers stems from a loss of meaning and empowerment in the therapeutic relationship, created (in part) as our chaotic healthcare system has shifted focus from quality issues to cost issues."

-David S. Jones and Sheila Quinn in *Textbook of Functional Medicine*

At this point, some of you may be saying, "Hey, our doctors and researchers are doing the best they can, and we just need to give them time to figure out how best to treat our epidemic of disease." I wish that were true. I wish that our insurance companies prioritized health over profit, that all medical research tried to find what actually causes disease and creates health, and that our education system taught doctors the best ways to eradicate chronic disease. Those things are not happening, and many doctors are frustrated when they realize that their training is inadequate when matched up with chronic disease.

By now you have probably guessed that I am highly critical of Western medicine, but I want to be clear: modern medicine can do miraculous things in an emergency. It can save lives when there is trauma and life-threatening infection, and it can slightly prolong life in end-stage chronic disease. However, when it comes to preventing and treating the chronic diseases that are becoming so ubiquitous in the U.S., the majority of our healthcare system is set up for failure. Because of the training doctors receive and the kinds of services insurance companies will pay for, people suffering from chronic disease don't stand a chance.

Our medical system has lost sight of what it means to be a doctor. The word "physician" is derived from the Greek word meaning "nature," and the word "doctor" is derived from the Latin word meaning, "to teach." I believe doctors are supposed to teach their patients how to achieve optimal health by helping them to align better with nature. Hippocrates, who is honored every time a medical school graduate takes the Hippocratic Oath to "first do no harm," said that a doctor "was to be skilled in Nature and must strive to know what man is in relation to food, drink, occupation, and which effect each of these has on the other." He would go on to say that a physician should never forget that disturbances in any organ correspond to a disturbance in the whole person, and to treat one organ you must address the whole person. As you will see in this chapter, I don't think Hippocrates would approve of the way medicine is being practiced today.

The Engine and Cost of "A Pill for an Ill"

A common occurrence in our healthcare system today goes like this: someone goes to their doctor with a complaint; the doctor diagnoses them, and then gives them a treatment. Seems simple enough, but the fact of the matter is far more complicated.

The doctor usually determines that a patient needs a certain type or length of treatment. However, the patient's insurance company may only pay for some or part of it. Wait a second—I thought that doctors went to medical school; aren't they the ones trained to determine the type and length of treatment, and shouldn't the insurance company be obligated to pay for what a doctor has deemed necessary? Regardless, this is the reality. Most people want to use the insurance they are spending so much money on and may not be able to pay out of pocket. So, even if the doctor thinks a patient would benefit more from a different treatment, they will tend to prescribe the treatment that they know the insurance company will cover. When it comes to chronic disease, insurance companies typically pay for the ineffective "pill for an ill" type of treatment and, unfortunately, since the doctors want to get paid, they tend to stick to that method, too.

Patients whose health would be better addressed in lifestyle medicine, nutritional medicine, or functional medicine will have to pay out of pocket for it. If they can't afford it, they're stuck with conventional medicine's pill. Medications don't fix the problem, they only mask symptoms, and eventually the patient ends up right back in the doctor's office with the same complaint or a new complaint that is a side effect of the original medication. This snowballs as treatments become increasingly aggressive—and expensive—and the patient worsens and possibly dies. The whole system caters to money rather than health.

I used to tell myself that one day insurance companies would figure out that paying for preventative care would save them more money in the long run. After all, paying for say, $5,000 worth of functional medicine to prevent a complicated disease, seems more cost effective than a lifetime of drugs or a $100,000 surgery. However, it was explained to me that when an insurance company has to pay for more expensive procedures for some, they are allowed to charge higher premiums to everyone because of their expenses. This means that insurance companies would rather pay for more expensive procedures, and lots of them, so they can make a bigger profit on premiums. The system is stacked against achieving proper healthcare.

Needless to say, the system is also proving costly. It is not only failing to stop many preventable deaths, it is also the leading cause of bankruptcy in this country. A Harvard study found that 62 percent of people who file for bankruptcy do so because they cannot afford the cost of medical treatment. A shocking 78 percent of those people had health insurance.[1] How sad is it that our healthcare is so expensive that it causes people to go bankrupt even if they have health insurance. Tragically, even after going bankrupt, many still don't get their health issues properly taken care of and many times end up sicker than when they started the medical treatments that caused the bankruptcy. What is really terrifying is that the total number of direct or indirect deaths attributed to the medical system is 793,936 per year, as reported by the 2011 health report, *Death by Medicine,* by Dr. Gary Null and others. That makes our healthcare system the leading cause of death in this country, even ahead of heart disease and cancer.

Why are we spending so much money on healthcare and getting such poor results? It may be that the system itself was not set up to achieve the health of patients, but rather for the profit of the healthcare system." In her book, *A Mind of Your Own,* Dr. Kelly Brogan states:

> After having witnessed the devastation this paradigm has wrought upon the lives of hundreds of my patients, I'm convinced that the pharmaceutical industry and its bedfellows, concealed behind official titles such as certain medical societies and associations, have created an illusion of science where none exists, in the service of profit over professional responsibility.

Neither she nor any other doctor that questions the Western medical model is a conspiracy theorist. She is coming to conclusions based on what she has observed working within the Western medical model. Patients don't get the treatment that will heal their bodies, they get medications that suppress symptoms and often cause more symptoms, which forces them back to the doctor for likely another medication. In this cycle, the doctors get rich, the insurance companies get rich, the pharmaceutical companies get rich, and the patients don't get better—many times they get much worse.

As of 2004, the United States ranks 37th in quality of health outcomes despite spending $1.6 trillion per year on healthcare, per the *Textbook of Functional Medicine*. That is way too much money to spend to be ranked that low in health outcomes. Those numbers make you wonder where all that money is going and if it is truly being used with patients in mind. It makes you question if time spent in the doctor's office is time well spent and worth paying for. If you are in the United States, you can just look around you every day and see the dismal outcomes of that $1.6 trillion.

Just like most everything in our capitalist society, medicine is a corporation. I have never run a corporation, nor do I want to, but if $1.6 trillion dollars a year was floating around in my company I would expect better results. If I didn't get them, I would stop investing—unless of course that investment was bringing in higher returns. Modern medicine is a business and it is in the business of "treating" disease. So what makes the industry more money, curing every disease it can until no one needs its services anymore, or creating treatments that don't address the real issue, only suppress symptoms—and very likely cause others—creating life-long repeat customers? It must be the latter, because I have never heard of a business offering such ineffective services becoming as economically successful as Medical Inc.

Looking back to the beginnings of our Western medical model, it clearly was never designed to work in the first place.

In his book, *Rockefeller Medicine Men,* E. Richard Brown tells us how the Western medicine model got started. Back in the late 1800s, a certain oil tycoon had just become extremely wealthy by pulling oil up out of the ground. Being the businessman that he was, John D. Rockefeller looked for ways to expand the uses of his abundance of oil. He hired scientists who discovered a way to use oil in the process of making pharmaceuticals; in fact, oil made the process much easier. With oil at their disposal his scientists found that they could more efficiently extract active ingredients out of a natural substance. Yes, the first pharmaceutical drugs were made with the help of substances in petroleum—talk about snake oil! Petroleum is still used in the making of many pharmaceuticals today.

Take Taxol for example. Taxol is a chemotherapy drug derived from the bark of the Pacific yew tree. Before petroleum came along it would have been difficult to extract the active ingredient from the bark. With petroleum it became much easier to get these extractions and made it possible to concentrate active ingredients into a pharmaceutical. The right extractions in the right concentrations could have desired effects on the body. Unfortunately, many of these extractions also come with nasty side effects. Taking Taxol usually come with hair loss, diarrhea, peripheral neuropathy, low blood counts, and vomiting. It amazes me that therapies with these kinds of side effects have become the standard of care in medicine. Rockefeller not only had a hand in developing these drugs but also in their rise to the top.

This oily man decided to do something about the many different types of healers who would compete with his products. In 1910, he hired a man to submit a report to Congress suggesting medicine needed standardization and oversight by an organization that would be the sole organization allowed to grant medical school licenses. Sadly, congress agreed, and that organization is now the

American Medical Association (AMA), which is built on the allopathic model of medicine—i.e. conventional medicine that prescribes drugs to target symptoms.

Since he had an abundance of money, Rockefeller then offered large grants to the best medical schools in the country, under the condition that their curriculum only teach the allopathic model. This man had suddenly gained massive control of medicine in the United States. He manufactured the only treatments and eliminated competitors. Those competitors have been fighting to remain afloat ever since. They persist mainly because there have always been people who value the effectiveness of approaches that exist outside of Western medicine. It is shocking to learn that at one point, in the 1960s, the AMA put together a committee whose job it was to put the profession of chiropractic out of commission. Luckily, they were unsuccessful.

I like to think that Mr. Rockefeller was not an evil man (at least, as far as I know) but just a driven and potentially single-minded businessman. As much as I hate some of the ways business is done in the world, discovering new uses for his material and eliminating competitors were profitable business decisions. Perhaps his actions were based on the best available understanding of disease and he thought he was doing good for mankind. The "pill for an ill" model could have been all the rage at the time. Had he known enough about how the body works and what people really need to be healthy, I like to think he would have done things differently, but that may be overly optimistic, and there are those who would disagree with me. Regardless, the history of the founding of the Western medical model explains a lot of why, and how, we got into the medical mess we are in today.

The Manipulation of Health Knowledge

I became disillusioned by Western medicine far before I learned how profit driven it is. It's been over 20 years since I was diagnosed with type 1 diabetes, and in that time, not a single endocrinologist mentioned any cause besides genetics. Not one of them told me that by changing my lifestyle, I could drastically decrease my use of insulin while maintaining an acceptable A1C level. I had to learn that by myself. Since I have been taking care of myself through lifestyle choices, my doctors have been perplexed at how well I am doing with my disease. One endocrinologist told me they didn't know what to do with me and insisted I retake thyroid tests to make sure other endocrine systems were okay. Another doctor tried to put me on a blood pressure medication to "protect" my kidneys, even though my blood pressure at the time of that office visit was 116/76 and my kidneys were showing no sign of decline. And I had a doctor try to put me on a cholesterol lowering statin drug because that is the standard of care for anyone who has been diabetic as long as I have. It is clear that these doctors are trained with one tool. They are legal drug dealers. I do not think my endocrinologists meant harm; however, I think they have been terribly misled by their medical education.

In medical school, we are not taught what creates optimum health in human beings. Rather, we learn basic anatomy and physiology, the classifying of symptoms, and the biochemical effects that drugs can have on those symptoms. In medical school there is no talk of health, no classes on the power of nutrition, and the curriculum and expectations are so demanding that many young doctors graduate in a state of poor health. More disheartening is the fact that most medical students start off wanting to help the sick and heal the world, but by the end they have been taught a medical model so focused on diagnostics that they refer to patients by their diseases instead of by their names.

Untrusty Research

Medical research, sadly, also does not escape the sickness of our system. I am not talking about the scientific method but rather the politics of research. If a researcher wants to conduct a study, they first and foremost need funding. The majority of medical research is funded by big pharmaceutical corporations because they have plenty of money and would like to have more research that validates their products. We owe much of what we know about the tiny biochemical reactions that happen in the body to the enormous amount of money that pharmaceutical companies have put into researching their products. However, due to the large cost, no pharmaceutical company is going to fund research without ensuring that the results will help them market their products, and so they fund studies with intentional bias. The conflict of interest is stunning. Tactics include designing studies to produce a desired outcome, playing with statistics to make a study appear more favorable than it is, and failing to publish studies that did not have the desired outcome.

Much of this kind of tampering has been exposed by Dr. Ben Goldacre, who has written about these concerning practices as well as the questionable results of pharmaceuticals. In his book, *Bad Science,* he illustrates that a much smaller majority of unfavorable studies end up getting published in medical journals, while the opposite is true for studies that produce the desired outcome. This is important because when a government agency is deciding whether they should approve a drug, they look to the medical literature. Let's say that exactly half of the research done on a particular drug yielded favorable results, and the other half unfavorable. Because journals are more likely to publish favorable results, then it is very likely that the governing body will see the results skewing favorable and may approve the drug never knowing that the entire research story has not been told. As Goldacre demonstrates, this is exactly what is happening. This can lead to the wrongful approval of drugs that are not safe, as was the case with the Merck & Co drug Vioxx, which resulted in the unnecessary deaths of tens of thousands of people by causing them to develop serious heart disease.

It's important to emphasize the influence these kinds of practices have in distorting the research appearing in medical journals. As a medical seeker-of-truth, when I search in the medical journals, I do not get an accurate representation of the collective body of research, because I can only access what has been selected for publication. This results in medical information that is misleading, unreliable to health practitioners, and potentially dangerous to patients.

It has also been demonstrated that many of the studies conducted for the purpose of getting a drug approved are not done for long enough duration in order to ensure safety. Many clinical trials last a few months and are then sent to the FDA for early approval because there have been no adverse effects. Many of these drugs get approved with only the knowledge that they are "safe" for short-term use. We have no idea if they are safe for long-term use, yet many patients are prescribed the medications for the long term anyway. Vioxx (used for arthritis and pain), Avandia (for blood sugar control), and the Premarin-progesterone hormone replacement combination are three examples of drugs that were tested short term and ended up causing disease or death to patients when taken long term. The sloppy work of these pharmaceutical companies for the sake of profit is costing lives.

As further evidence that our healthcare system is driven by money, the treatments recommended to patients by providers are largely influenced by pharmaceutical and insurance companies. Doctors get much of their on-the-job training about new drugs from representatives of pharmaceutical companies who have little biomedical science background. Since doctors are not well equipped to handle chronic disease without medications, they are dependent on these pharmaceutical representatives for new treatments. The representatives bring lunch and teach doctors how new drugs work. Given the fact that the representatives and their companies benefit if doctors prescribe the drug, there is a huge conflict of interest. It is not uncommon for doctors to get bonuses from companies for reaching certain prescribing goals. Many sketchy things could go wrong here. The representative could emphasize the positive research and neglect the negative research when trying to sell to the doctor, they could push the most expensive drugs rather than the safest or most effective, and the doctor could prescribe a drug to someone who may not necessarily need it because of a desire for a kickback from the pharmaceutical company. All this is going on without the interest of the patient in mind.

Even if we could eliminate these extreme biases, there is another more core philosophical issue I take with the way in which research is conducted. Let's step back and look at research with a wider lens. In my opinion, research is flawed at a fundamental level. The highest quality research is considered to be a randomized, double blind, placebo-controlled trial. This type of study is one where many different variables are eliminated in order to isolate a single product or procedure. The argument is that this isolation guarantees that product or procedure caused the outcome of the study. For chronic disease, this is flawed thinking. Hippocrates stressed the emphasis of treating the body as a whole and not just one biochemical pathway. Rarely—if ever—are humans affected by only a single isolated stimulus that affects a single isolated biochemical pathway. So in some cases, a more productive way of doing research would be to see if certain combinations of stimuli that we are experiencing in our modern lives are having an effect on our health. A perfect example of this is the research being done to see if there is any link between vaccines and autism. If we keep trying to design research to see if vaccines single handedly cause autism then the collective body of research will continue to give us a "definitely maybe not" answer. However, if we started to study whether the combination of things like children not being natural births, not being breast-fed, and eating food that has been sprayed with herbicides like glyphosate in conjunction with the increased vaccine schedules, then I think we will start to get real answers to the question of what is behind the increase in autism, or any of the other chronic diseases on the rise.

Shifting Paradigms

As a species, we have been questioning our ways of living and our understanding of the body from long before Western medicine came into the picture. As one example, the late 19th century Austrian philosopher, Rudolf Steiner, stated that there are three important ideological changes necessary for humans to continue evolving: people need to stop working for money, to realize there is no difference between sensory and motor nerves, and to understand that the heart is not a pump. Steiner's ideas may seem heretical but their underlying philosophical suggestion plays well into the theme of this book: if we want to progress as a species, then our modern understandings of human nature, biology, and health are in need of an upgrade.

This goes back to Chapter 2: How can we go to our doctor today and be given a clean bill of health despite being very unhealthy and struggling through each and every day? Steiner hints at conventional wisdoms that need to be rethought, but what we really need is an entirely different framework to measure health, because the framework modern medicine has given us is not cutting it and has led us astray in many other aspects of health as well.

A perfect example of this can be found in our public health system. Public health programs rarely address more pressing health issues because they focus on the profitable "pill for an ill" philosophy pushed by Medical Incorporated. In his book, *Human Heart, Cosmic Heart,* Dr. Thomas Cowan illustrates some of what I mean:

> Eight percent of prisoners worldwide are African American men imprisoned in the United States. Might this be a larger health problem for African American communities than cholesterol levels? The main cause of death for children living in the Gaza Strip is war-related trauma. Might this be a comparable, or larger, public health issue than whether they are vaccinated against measles? Every drop of mother's milk, human or animal, on the entire planet is contaminated with toxic and carcinogenic chemicals. Are we to believe that group B strep in the birth canal or hepatitis B injections within hours after birth are a more important intervention than a public health initiative to make sure these types of chemicals never show up in our mothers' milk?

The pills, vaccines, and injections mentioned above are important, but by correcting the reductive way healthcare has been defined in this nation, I believe we could find endless examples of dire public health issues that are overlooked.

Another of medicine's blunders—perhaps its largest—is its failure to account for the fact that humans are a product of millions of years of evolving along with our natural environment. Since

Western medicine was developed only in the last century, every lab test, examination, and procedure conducted has been on humans who are removed from the environment in which they evolved. One result of this is that the "normal" ranges of lab tests and procedures that your doctor gives you are based on modern-day humans. Imagine taking a group of giraffes, breeding them in captivity, and feeding them an unnatural diet of McDonalds and Chinese takeout for many generations. The health and disease markers for those giraffes would be very different from wild ones, and basing the standard for giraffe health on those captive animals would be shortsighted at best. Research even indicates that normal health marker ranges in people who live a more traditional lifestyle are different from those of us who are living a standard Western lifestyle.[2,3]

You can see how that person considered "generally healthy" in Chapter 2 could be misled even by their bloodwork, which is based on these normal ranges for Westernized people. Shouldn't we be more focused on achieving lab numbers comparable to people who live in their natural environment and are free of chronic disease? Further, a multitude of research is now showing how wrong the cholesterol theory of heart disease was and how good the right types of saturated fat can be for us. This forces us to confront the fact that the last 60 years of developing treatments for heart disease based on that theory (statins, stents, and bypass surgeries) have all been based on incorrect information. Makes you wonder what else we got wrong about disease.

Sigh. It is easy to get sucked into a rabbit hole of negativity when talking about the shortcomings of our medical system. When this happens, I try to step back and force myself to think positively. I tell myself that the profit-driven companies controlling our healthcare system are operated through the work of good people stuck in a bad system. I have to remind myself that these people are just working to ensure they have what they need to survive. Many people, even if they don't believe in what their employer does or even if they see a major ethical violation, are inclined to keep their heads down solely because they have themselves and maybe a family to support. No one can blame them; this is just how society is set up. As Upton Sinclair said, "It is difficult to get a man to understand something, when his salary depends on his not understanding it." This is why I don't like to blame the problems of our health care on the so-called evil, money-driven CEOs running companies, even if that really is the way they are. I like to think that humans are just selfishly programmed beings stuck in a profit-driven society. It is a bad combination and it isn't necessarily any one person's fault. Michael Crichton sums this up well in his book, *Travels.* He addresses a group of friends who have been blaming "them" for many of society's problems. He points out to his friends that there isn't any "they" but only people like you and me. If a CEO looks like a jerk while trying to explain a questionable action his company has been accused of, he is probably dealing with issues at home or unreliable employees or a dysfunctional work environment just like many of us do. Crichton also says that even if CEOs and corporations are evil, it still doesn't make sense to blame *them:*

> What's really wrong with making *them* the problem is that you abdicate your own responsibility. Once you say some mysterious *they* are in charge then you're able to sit back comfortably and complain about how *they* are doing it. But maybe *they* need your help. Maybe *they* need your ideas and your support and your letters and your active participation. Because you're not powerless, you are a participant in this world. It's your world, too.

We see here that the answer, at least to an individual's sanity, is to stop blaming others for the problems of healthcare, and of the world, and start realizing that the real issue is that our society is set up in a way that makes it hard for some people to keep their jobs in order to support their family without making some questionable decisions during their career. Another way to phrase all of this is don't hate the player, hate the game. The big problem is that we all just sit back and live the life that society creates for us without questioning it. Our current healthcare system is just one aspect of society that is affected by our failure to question our capitalist system. When it comes to medicine, especially since changes in any science are hard to come by, sitting back and blaming others will only make the process of changing medicine even harder than it already is.

So what can we do?

In *The Structure of Scientific Revolutions*, Thomas Khun warns us that "changes of 'normative' science rarely come from within," which tells us that we cannot rely on conventional medicine to acknowledge its short comings and take steps to change them. This is demonstrated in the story of the Hungarian physician Ignaz Semmelwies. In the 1850s, while at the University of Vienna, he discovered that the unwashed hands of doctors delivering babies was causing fatal infections among new mothers. When he aggressively came forward with this notion, which we now know is true, he was stripped of his medical license, removed from his academic position at the school, and eventually died disgraced. New ideas in science are not always welcomed with open arms. One reason for this could be because there are those out there whose life work depends on the old ideas and they see new ideas as a threat to their careers.

The physicist Max Planck enlightens us with the realization that science is more political than we think:

> A new scientific truth does not triumph by convincing its opponents and making them see the light, but rather because its opponents die, and a new generation grows up that is familiar with it.

This is the same for Western medicine. I believe that instead of telling those practicing modern medicine that they are wrong, we must teach the next generation of healers a new approach to health. This starts with an overhaul in medical school curriculum. That process could be a very long and politically challenging one.

In the meantime, if we want to see a change in how medicine is practiced and how medical research is done then we need to demand a better product. Adding to the words of Crichton, I would say maybe *they* need to see a demand for better-trained doctors. As patients we need to demand better results by seeking out practitioners that know how to achieve positive health results and not just the suppression of symptoms. Medicine is a business with a product, and if consumers demand different products the business has no choice but to respond. We'll discuss how to demand a better product by finding better practitioners in Chapter 16.

As a society we seem to not understand where health comes from at all. It can be paralyzing to recognize that our rates of chronic disease are spiraling out of control, our healthcare system is not well equipped to handle it, and our capitalist society is holding back objective progress. If you feel, however, that the conclusion is that we are doomed, I hope you continue reading. While I enjoy keeping up with the latest research and continue to be amazed at human ingenuity, I personally feel that the answer to our health woes lies in the careful investigation of the past and not in the science of the future. The coming pages will unravel the mystery of chronic disease in humans and how we can achieve positive health results, but first we need to understand how we got into this mess. This will require a headfirst dive into something that has remained constant since the beginning of life on the planet: evolution.

Part Two: The Evolutionary Explanation

Chapter 5: My College Evolution

I was startled awake by the sounds of books closing and students shuffling out of their seats. Class was over. I was thankful to be in the largest lecture hall at my alma mater, the University of North Carolina Asheville, because that most likely meant the professor hadn't noticed me sleeping. It was unlike me to sleep in class. I have always been a rule follower and really did value my education, but as a freshman in college, I had no passion, and it just felt like no matter how early I went to bed I was always so tired.

The complete lack of emotion from Dr. Peters lecturing at the front of the room didn't help either. After you got over the fluffy hair and oversized glasses that made him look like he was stuck in the eighties, his monotone lectures were sure to put you to sleep.

Everyone told me that the sciences were the hardest classes for an incoming freshman, but I had liked my pediatric endocrinologist so much that it inspired me to go the pre-med route. Ecology and Evolution was first on the pre-med checklist, along with biology and chemistry. But I soon got a wake-up call. High school had been easy and I rarely had to study, but now I was almost through my first semester and both biology and chemistry were really handing it to me. Despite memorizing my study sheets and having friends quiz me, I would get into the tests feeling like I must have studied the wrong material. I wasn't prepared for college-level courses.

I remember requesting a meeting with my Ecology and Evolution lab instructor to discuss how I should study. After giving me study tips and resources to learn the material she put her hand on my shoulder and said, "Stephen, you have to find the subject that drives you to learn more; you have to really love it." I left that meeting freaking out a little because I felt that biology and chemistry were not something I really loved, and I was failing both.

That first year was hell. I flirted with academic probation just long enough to finally find something I was passionate about: health. It makes sense considering all the health issues I had experienced. With a quick change of major, things started looking up for me—applying biology was simple once I focused it on human health. I remember having to do a project for nutrition class on the effects that vitamins and minerals have on our health and soon found that this had major overlap with my chemistry classes. Assessing cardiovascular health markers in my health classes made learning about the physiology of the heart in biology classes that much more applicable. Intermixing classes in the sciences and in health promotion was exactly what I needed to get through college, and it sent me on a quest to determine what was happening with my health.

Things would come full circle in such an ironic way. I nearly failed my first course in evolution, but it wasn't until I could see the world through that lens that I found the health answers I was looking for.

Chapter 6: A Crash Course in Evolution

"Nothing in biology makes sense except in the light of evolution."

-Theodosius Dobzhansky

Evolution is one of the most important discoveries the human species has ever made. It has allowed us to better understand the natural world and our place in it. Studying the history of humans in the context of evolution could do amazing things if we let it. For example, it has shown us that we all came from the same descendants, and we are all 99.9% alike. Perhaps when we see people as different because of their race, religion, or creed, we can use this information as a reminder that many times we should focus on how remarkably alike we all are. Studying human evolution has also revealed that it would have been nearly impossible to evolve the brains we have today without the consumption of animal fat and meats and that they are essential for our health. With this information perhaps we can focus our efforts on finding ways to raise animals in ways that are humane, sustainable, and regenerative rather than wasting time, energy, and money debating whether or not we should eat animals. When it comes to predicting the future of our planet—and what we can do to ensure humans are included in that future—evolutionary science has the potential to be the most influential of the sciences.

Evolution entered the general body of scientific knowledge around 1859 when Darwin published his seminal book, *On the Origins of Species.* Humans have known about evolution for less than 200 years and it has already opened so many new doors of knowledge. Conversely, it seems we haven't reckoned with its fullest implications. It's time to let it guide us to explanations for the health crisis we are in. First, we need to set a foundation on the basics of evolution.

Evolution is at the core of life on this planet. It is "survival of the fittest," as is popularly said. Yet, from an evolutionary perspective, "fittest" doesn't necessarily mean biggest, strongest, fastest, or healthiest. On the contrary—fitness is entirely dependent on the environment the living thing happens to be in. In the textbook, *Principles of Evolutionary Medicine,* the environment of an organism is defined as "the sum of all the external conditions and stimuli that it experiences, including climate, nutrient supply, social structure resulting from other members of its own species, and threats from other species in the form of predation, parasitism, or infection." To illustrate how these contribute to fitness, let's focus in on access to food. Imagine that we put chimpanzees and horses in a single isolated environment. In this environment, the only food available is in trees. Obviously, the chimps are fit for this environment, but the horses have a high likelihood of starving. Switching things up, let's add a small predator to the mix and say that the only food available is on the ground. Great for the horses who can eat the food and are too big for the predators to threaten, but the monkeys are now suddenly at a disadvantage as they have to take the risk of coming down to the ground to eat. This is a vastly oversimplified example, but I hope it demonstrates well how our environment determines the fitness of an individual.

As I said, a common misconception that people make is that fittest means the strongest, fastest, prettiest, and smartest individuals are the ones that survive—traits many of us are certainly obsessed with as a species. As the previous example shows, while those characteristics can help in some situations, it is only those individuals with characteristics best suited for their environment that will win the evolutionary game of passing on their genes. Modern society is reluctant to apply evolution to humans. Perhaps it is because we are taught that we must choose between evolution and creationism, or maybe it is because we want to see ourselves as separate from nature. Whatever the reason, evolution has implications that are necessary for our survival, and so it is high time that we allow ourselves to see humans through an evolutionary lens. There are four concepts about evolution that I want to go over and then I will demonstrate how it explains our health crisis in Chapter 8. These are concepts that, when I first learned them, sparked *a-ha* moments of life-changing realization.

The first concept is "natural selection," the process by which living things evolve in relationship to their environment. I used to find it so hard to fathom how a living thing could physically change one of its characteristics in order to pass on better genes. Turns out I couldn't imagine that because that is not what happens! In order for a species to evolve, first the selection pressures around it have to change. This change causes certain less "fit" members of any particular species to die, ensuring their "unfit" genes don't get passed on. The genes of those best suited for the environment do get passed on, and their offspring create a new generation possessing those same genes. Evolution is not a conscious thought process; it is a dynamic interaction between the environment and living things. As humans, it is hard for us to imagine such a powerful and influential force that operates unconsciously, because everything about individual human life is experienced through conscious thought. But evolution is an unconscious force, an unavoidable law of nature, just as magnetism is an unavoidable law of physics. Let me explain.

Looking at our former simplistic example, let's introduce food scarcity into the first scenario. By a random coincidence of nature—just as some humans are taller and some are shorter—some of the monkeys were born with longer tails that made them better at climbing in trees. The monkeys with shorter tails will fail to get food more often, and over time will die off, while the longer-tailed monkeys will thrive, reproduce, and create a new generation of solely long-tailed monkeys. When this sort of thing happens vastly over many generations, it can lead to animals that look entirely different from that original monkey. Different individuals of the same species can be greatly affected when variations in physical characteristics create unequal competition in a given environment.

We can see small evolutionary changes in the animal kingdom occurring today—for example, tree-dwelling lizards with newly extra sticky feet that let them outcompete other lizards, stealthy owls whose feathers have changed color along with their changing environment, and mice that have become immune to our poisons. However, larger, species-level changes occur over so many generations that we will never see this kind of drastic evolutionary change happen in a single lifetime.

Natural selection is a fascinatingly complex process, with many varying types of pressure interacting to evolve life. One of those pressures, a special type of natural selection, is sexual selection. A classic example of sexual selection is the peacock. Male peacocks have developed extravagant tail feathers to impress peahens and increase the chances that they will be selected as mates and pass on their genes. Extravagant feathers demonstrate that the peacocks are healthy, have good genes, and are quick enough to evade predators despite having the equivalent of a neon "edible prey" sign on their backside—all qualities that females desire for their offspring. Over time the peahens select the peacocks with the best tail feathers and those genes get passed on until all peacocks have these impressive displays. Still, some are more impressive than others and the competition goes on. When you understand this process, you can start to flesh out the many curious characteristics of living beings, both human and animal, and it becomes fun to wonder what selection pressures resulted in the life we see all around us today.

Another phenomenon that drives natural selection is random genetic mutation that occurs as genes are passed on. Darwin's famous example is that of the Galapagos finches and their beaks. Occasionally a finch was born with a slightly different beak than others of his species, simply due to a random genetic mutation. If this mutation was favorable, meaning it improved that finch's ability to survive by, say, letting it gain access to food better than his peers, then this finch would have a greater chance of passing on his mutated, advantageous beak genes. This finch's offspring would have that same advantage, would out-compete others and pass on those same genes. Eventually, all the members of that species would have the advantageous genes. Some mutations play out so well that they can become a trademark of a species, like the long ant-catching tongue of an anteater. The opposite, where a mutation occurs that leaves the offspring at a disadvantage, can happen as well, though they will be out-competed and their disadvantageous genes won't be seen or heard from too much down the road. In *On the Origin of Species* Darwin sums up mutation:

> Whatever the cause may be of each slight difference in
> the offspring from their parents—and cause for each

must exist—it is the steady accumulation, through natural selection, of such differences, when beneficial to the individual, that gives rise to all the more important modifications of structure, by which the innumerable beings on the face of this earth are enabled to struggle with each other, and the best adapted to survive.

These three examples of food scarcity for monkeys, peahens mating based on tail feathers, and random genetic mutations of beaks simplify evolution for the sake of illustrating what kinds of pressures drive evolution. In reality, evolution happens with many, many types of selection pressures acting on living things all at once. Evolutionary scientists have the challenging task of deducing which selection pressures produced the many characteristics of species we see today. The big idea to grasp is that species evolve as a whole, and in order for evolution to take place the genes of less fit individuals must not be passed on and the genes of more fit individuals must survive. If you still can't quite wrap your head around evolution, the third evolutionary concept might shed some light on why it's so hard for us to grasp, but first let's clear up the misconception that humans evolved from apes.

The second concept we need to understand is that human beings are still subject to evolution. To provide an example of how we are a part of evolution and to clear up a common misconception, let's look to the past.

Many people think evolution insists that we evolved from chimpanzees, our closest living ancestor. Personally, I like to think I descended from a big, strong, handsome gorilla. Unfortunately, both of these ideas fall prey to an incorrect line of thinking. Humans did not evolve from apes. Rather, humans and apes share a common ancestor. The species of apes alive today probably didn't exist in distant history, just as modern humans didn't. What did exist was a living being that both modern day apes and humans evolved from. Who knows what it looked like or what we would have called it, but since we both came from it and I think it's fun, I'm going to call it a "hape."

If you're having doubts here, please bear with me and know that there's extensive and ever-expanding hard evidence (i.e. the fossil record) of common ancestors evolving into modern humans and apes over large spans of time. This isn't "theory" in the sense of "a possible idea," but "theory" in the sense of Einstein's Theory of General Relativity. As the gaps in the fossil record continue to be filled, our material understanding of our connectedness to other species, both living and extinct, will only continue to grow.

So how did two very different species evolve from the same ancestors? Well, imagine a group of hapes just living and doing their thing. One day half of the group decides to up and leave, or maybe some natural disaster forces the group to split apart. We now have two hape populations living in two different parts of the world that vary in climate, terrain, and ultimately selection pressures. Over time these differing pressures push the groups in two evolutionary directions. Along the way to humans and apes, there were many mutations and even other species that developed and branched off from the two groups. They rose, played a part in this extremely long evolutionary process, and fell. We have recovered remains of some of these branch-off species, like Australopithecus africanus, Homo habilis, and Homo erectus. We may never know for sure what allowed modern humans to out-compete all the other variations, but here we are. So we did not evolve from apes, but apes and humans evolved from a common progenitor. That split happened around an estimated 6 million years ago and demonstrates that we humans are, too, the result of, and still subject to, evolution.

The third evolutionary concept will help you wrap your head around the first two a bit better. This concept is that evolutionary change takes a very long time (think of *The Sandlot:* "Foooor-eeeev-eeeer"), so long that we really have to step back and marvel at the expanse of it. It's hard for us to grasp something so vastly longer than a single human lifetime. In the words of Darwin, "We see nothing of these slow changes in progress, until the hand of time has marked the long lapses of ages, and then so imperfect is our view into long past geological ages, that we only see that the forms of life are now different from what they formally were." However, human ingenuity never ceases to amaze me—in an attempt to see evolution in progress, one Russian scientist conducted some amazing work.

In 1959, Dimitry Belyaev began an experiment in which he started selectively breeding wild red foxes for tame traits to see if he could essentially domesticate them. Who wouldn't want a pet fox? To do this he only allowed the male and female foxes that displayed more docile behavior to breed. He did this generation after generation. After about 30 generations (foxes reproduce far faster than humans), he realized that not only were the foxes acting almost like domesticated dogs but that certain physical characteristics (ears, tails, fur) were changing. This happened because they did not need those characteristics for survival in the wild anymore, and it became evolutionarily advantageous to display the tame, cute and cuddly traits that humans desire. This is the same thing that humans have done, intentionally or unintentionally, with cows, horses, sheep, pigs, cats, dogs, camels, and llamas. Tentatively, Belyaev showed that it takes at least 30 generations for life to show signs of evolutionary change. Sadly, Belyaev died in 1985, but others are continuing his work and I believe they are nearing the 50th generation of fox-dogs. Doxes? Fogs? Either way, they are man's best sly friend.

Now, despite it taking only 30 generations to changes these foxes, we cannot say that 30 generations is the standard for life to show evolutionary change. Belyaev may have gotten physical and behavioral changes in 30 generations, but he did it with very controlled domestic breeding. In nature this would have been happening with multiple factors guiding favorable traits. It wouldn't be as cut and dried as Balyaev's experiments.

Based on Balyaev's 30 generations estimate and the fact that a human generation is loosely 25 years, it would take an extreme minimum 750 years to see substantive, sustained change in humans. I don't know about you, but I don't have a very good idea what humans looked like that long ago. I don't even know what my great-great-grandparents looked like, and that was only four generations ago. When I see depictions of earlier humans in cave drawings from tens of thousands of years ago or in ancient art, I often think they look a little different from the humans I see around me today. I used to chalk it up to the fact that ancient artists weren't as good as artists are today, but who knows? Maybe humans just looked slightly different way back then. This idea is complete speculation, but it's fun to think about.

I wish the photograph had been invented 500 generations ago, roughly the time that humans went through a substantial lifestyle change that we will discuss in the next chapter. I'd love to see how similar—or, more intriguingly, how different—our ancestors' appearance was to our own. It will be incredible when generations of genetic humans far in the future look at the first photographs of humans and say, "They look a lot different than we do today." The take home is that evolution happens over such a large amount of time that it is hard for us to grasp the grandness of it all. It is not something that we see happening on a day-to-day—or even century-to-century—timescale.

It is such a large concept I feel that many people believe that we are an end point of evolution—the culmination of life. If they had had our same quantity of knowledge, I bet every ancestral species that came before us would have felt the same way. The point, to return to our third concept, is that even though it may not seem like it, in reality we are still susceptible to evolution. It's hard to see this possibility when we have only been able to record history for about 5,500 years. One million years from now who knows if humans will still look and behave like we do. Maybe we will evolve so drastically, we won't even be the same species.

I have saved the concept most important to my argument for last. After this principle, you may start to see where this book is going. Life is intricately connected to the environment in which it grows. Because of this, survival can be a very fragile thing for an individual, and even for an individual species. Living things migrate, kill, learn new behaviors, eat new foods, and do just about whatever they have to do to survive. Through the passing on of "fit" genes, complex living beings have survived ever-changing selection pressures for the 600 million years that multi-cellular life has been on Earth. In other words, life is also incredibly resilient, and it is the diversity and adaptability of life that makes it so resilient. There are situations in which forms of life are very fragile, and Earth has seen these situations a number of times. If a species finds itself in the midst of one of these circumstances and is not well equipped to handle the changes, then no matter how hard the individuals of that species may try, they won't make it.

In *The Sixth Extinction,* Elizabeth Kolbert says, "A species that needs to migrate to keep up with rising temperatures, but is trapped in a forest fragment—even a very large forest fragment—is a species that isn't likely to make it." When some unforeseen, drastic environmental event happens quickly enough, it is really hard for any species to produce the necessary generations needed to adapt. Kolbert points out that there have been five major extinctions in the history of life on Earth in which large quantities of living beings died off. Each of these extinctions was preceded by massive global changes. She warns that humans are creating the conditions for—and are likely in the middle of—the 6th extinction.

We are now losing species at the rate of one per day. If you're asking yourself why there is concern over such accelerated loss, I'll remind you that as different as we seem from life in the natural world, and as far removed from the natural world as we have made ourselves, we are still a part of it. Changes that happen in the natural world affect us, too.

I see an echo between this and medication's impact on the body. Medications do not create health, and cause numerous side effects, because they are designed to affect one biochemical pathway to get a desired result. But the body is a complex network of many biochemical interactions, many of which we still don't understand or even know about. It's foolish to think we can isolate one desired pathway with a medication. Biochemical interactions are so complex and interconnected that altering one is inevitably going to impact many others, and because we may never fully understand the workings of the body, the side effects that come from altered biochemical reactions are almost impossible to predict. The same is true with our natural world. Every species plays a critical part in the environment we have all co-evolved in for millions of years. What happens when enough species, or one group of very important species like pollinators, becomes extinct and leaves a void in the natural maintenance of our environment? Will this void (or another void) affect the planet's ecosystem to such an extent that sustenance is jeopardized for other species? And if more species, in turn, go extinct, where does that leave us? Will the world change enough that it starts the process of our own extinction? Will it then be too late for us to do something about it?

Like the infamous canary in the coalmine, our chronic disease epidemic is a warning sign that something in evolution has gone awry. When addressing the question of why natural selection has not rescued our bodies from being so vulnerable to these kinds of disease, the textbook, *Principles of Evolutionary Medicine,* gives us three possible answers:

> First, evolution is too slow and cannot cope with either the co-evolutionary microbiotic arms race or with novel environments, especially those of human making. Second, there are constraints on what selection can do and often there are inevitable trade-offs which themselves have consequences. Third, there may be consequences to what selection has shaped because selection is about fitness not health.

The point I want to emphasize is that although evolution is an ingenious way for nature to respond to the ever-changing planet Earth, it is not a way to ensure the continuation of one species or another. It doesn't ensure the health of any individual within a species, only life as a whole. When changes happen too quickly, living things don't stand a chance—especially living things with very long reproduction cycles, like ours.

This is the fourth and final concept, the most important thing I have taken from outside the medical field and applied to health: *when the environment of an individual changes too rapidly, it is very difficult for that being to maintain health and survive.* However, humans have evolved a famous trademark characteristic—a very large brain. Instead of adapting with nature, humans began to *adapt nature* on a large scale. Most of life is a delicate balance of symbiotic give and take, with built-in fail-safes in case any one species begins to drain an ecosystem. Because of human ingenuity, however, we have found ways to sustain ourselves while simultaneously draining the resources around us. In the next couple of chapters, and especially in Chapter 8, we'll take a closer look at this final principle. When I understood it, it was like the clouds parting. The cause of our disease epidemic became so clear.

Chapter 7: An Unexpected Treasure Hunt in Paradise

ooking down at the boat, I did not get a reassuring feeling. It reminded me a little too much of the beat-up skiff on the church playground where we kids used to pretend we were sailing the high seas. That boat was in no condition to sail anywhere and the one I was now riding in made me wish I was back on the playground. With every bump the boat let out a creak of complaint.

Looking up and out, the scene was a bit more pleasant. We had just left the mainland of Panama and were on our way to San Blas, an archipelago of approximately 365 tropical islands in the Caribbean. I had just begun a three-and-a-half month backpacking trip through Central America with my roommate, and this was one of our first adventures. After riding in Jeeps through the jungle all morning, we had boarded these "boats" to our final destination.

The view was stunning. I had never been to a place like this. The sea was a clear teal and the islands were just little collections of palm trees scattered about. As we approached the island where we would be staying, it couldn't have looked more idyllic. The island could probably be traversed in a mere five minutes on foot. Our hosts were two young Panamanian men. As I explored our new digs I realized that for the next few days I would essentially be outside—the only structures around were huts. Camping on the beach sounded good to me. There were also a few families of the indigenous Guna people on the island.

Unfortunately, my stay was not all stress-free living. On the very first day I was playing Frisbee on the beach with a young Australian woman who was also staying on the island. Both being amateur Frisbee-ers, sometimes our throws were a little off target and we would have to run into the ocean to try and catch it. There were times where I had to go deeper into the surf to retrieve the Frisbee and it wasn't until about the third time that I realized I still had my insulin pump in my pocket. I quickly tugged it out to inspect it and, to my horror, I could see that there was water in the display screen. I pushed a few buttons to see if it worked, and it gave me error messages. This was not good.

Luckily, my mother, forward thinking person that she is, had recommended that I request a travel pump from the company in case I needed it while gallivanting through Central America. There was one problem. When replacing the batteries in these pumps or putting a battery in for the first time, it has to be a completely new battery, which I had left with my other belongings back at the main hostel in Panama City. Here I was on a secluded island, among islands with no electricity and few battery-powered electronics. It was at least a half-day's journey back to anywhere there might be batteries. My Australian Frisbee partner, my roommate, and I were the only ones staying there at the time and none of us had any batteries. The boat that we came in on had already left for the evening, and I was starting to realize that this was going to be a very long and uncomfortable night.

While high blood sugar is not as dangerous short term as low blood sugar, I was all too familiar with how terrible it would make me feel and the damage it would cause if left unchecked. I hurried over to our two young hosts, with whom I could not talk because I did not speak Spanish, and somehow communicated that I desperately needed a battery. They seemed to have an idea.

They guided me around a small bluff of the island to a boat. It was smaller and looked just as unsafe as the last one, but I didn't care at this point. I was hoping that they knew of a nearby 7/11. I had no idea if they knew exactly what I needed or where they thought we were going to find it, but I hopped in. After about five minutes of riding out from the island and passing other small, uninhabited islands, I saw an island in the distance that looked different from the others. It had far fewer trees on it. Once we got closer I could see that this island was completely covered with little huts—it was a little village.

Our arrival disrupted a game of soccer being played in an area no bigger than a basketball court. As I stepped onto shore the players surrounded me in interest. In my haste to find a battery I hadn't put on a shirt when leaving the other island, and one man who greeted us gave me a concerned look, disappeared into a hut, and came out with a shirt for me to put on. My two guides then waved for me to follow them, and we walked through the village.

I was shocked at how my surroundings had changed. Beside the fact that it did not look like a place to find a battery, I had gone from tropical paradise to what looked like a poverty-stricken village. The people were very curious about me, and some kids kept kicking a small soccer ball toward me and were excited when I kicked back and played a little keep away.

The huts were built out of what looked like small tree trunks lined up next to each other, and they were packed tightly, side-by-side, creating little through-ways like streets. I caught a few glimpses inside some of the huts and could see that these people didn't have much. Most of the huts had dirt floors, little cot-like beds, and small makeshift kitchens. One hut in particular was larger than the others and seemed to be a place where people of the village gathered. At this particular moment there was lots of smoke coming from the doors of the hut and there were about 20 people kneeling in the room. I was so busy taking in all the things around me that I almost completely forgot about my battery.

I was brought back to reality by a tug on my borrowed shirtsleeve. One of my guides was pointing to a door. He walked me over and knocked on it. The door didn't open, but a little window that was next to it did. Inside, it was lined like a convenience store from a world very far from my own. I saw bags of Doritos, hand-held radios, little boxes of Cheez-Its, bottled water, tape, and...batteries! It was like I had found a lost buried treasure chest. All I had on me was my swim suit and someone else's shirt, so I had no money, but one of my hosts bought me a pack and gave me a thumbs up. I was saved. We went back to the boat a different way through the village, I returned the shirt, and we took off back to our island.

On the way back, I thought about how, despite having Cheez-Its at their disposal, the islanders still hunted and gathered from the environment. The quote by Robin Williams kept running through my head: *We used to be hunter-gatherers, now we're shopper-borrowers*. These people were a little of both. I wondered if they were ever faced with situations like mine. Were they that reliant on something like a battery? Did they even get diabetes? I also thought about how our ancient ancestors used to have to hunt for what they needed to survive and how in this situation I was sort of hunting for what I needed to survive. It's funny to think about the different objects of our hunts—a wildebeest vs. a battery. These thoughts lasted until we arrived back to our island. With the crisis averted the rest of the evening was spent by a fire on the beach laughing about how close a call that was. Finally, I could return to enjoying the travel—or so I thought.

The next day around three or four I saw our two hosts head out into the surf with their spears. I had seen them do this at various times since we had arrived. They were catching the food that they had been feeding us. Talk about fresh! The spears they used were sharpened sticks with an elastic-like cord attached to the dull end. The loose end of the cord had a loop in it which was supposed to go around your wrist. Once around your wrist you would stretch the cord enough so that you could grab close to the sharp end of the spear. When you found something worth spearing you would let go of the spear and the tension on the cord would dart it through the water and hopefully hit your next meal.

Lucky for me they had left an extra spear on the beach, and I decided to try my luck in the shallow areas, being sure to leave my insulin pump on land this time. I soon found out that fishing like this was pretty much impossible, at least for me. It turned out to be very difficult to hold the spear with tension on the cord for any more than 10-15 seconds before my arm got painfully fatigued. And when I did let go, aiming was a whole other story. The water was so clear that when I was under I could see our two hosts further out in the ocean over a bed of coral surrounding the island. They would keep freediving down near the coral, let the spear fly, come back up, and then try again until they got something. I decided to venture out over the coral.

It was beautiful. The colors were mesmerizing and there were so many kinds of life to appreciate. At this point the surface of the water was about 5-6 feet above the coral and I was swimming around in those 5-6 feet of water. At one point my goggles and snorkel got some water in them and I surfaced to get everything situated. While I was treading water my foot must have hit the coral below me because I felt a sudden sharp stinging pain in my right heel. I put my goggles on and looked under the water to see a red scrape on my heel and streams of blood disappearing into the water.

Having seen too many movies, I made a B-line for shore out of pure fear of sharks hunting me down. I arrived exhausted. My roommate came over to see what was up. In all this excitement I didn't see that our hosts were back with our dinner. They joined the huddle around me, looked at my heel, and made wincing faces. My roommate had her Spanish book with her and I told her to look up the word for shark. When she said it our two hosts immediately cracked up. I didn't know why at that moment but I found out later that the only sharks in these waters would have been nurse sharks, and they were nothing to worry about. At least I had given them a laugh.

After dinner, my heel was very tender and swollen even walking in the soft white sand. I cleaned my cut in the ocean and then hopped on one foot back to my hut and turned in for the night. I awoke at about two in the morning with severe pain in my heel. It was throbbing. This trip was my much-deserved break at my halfway point through chiropractic school. I had just learned a ton about basic sciences and diagnosis, but all I could think about at the moment was cellulitis and how quickly it could turn into a life-threatening situation.

It was a painful and restless night. I just stared through some holes in the palm leaves roof of my hut for what seemed like forever. The full moon was huge. I decided to go and soak my foot in the ocean again. I took my headlamp, but when I got outside I realized I didn't need it. The ocean and the sand were reflecting the moon so brilliantly that it almost felt like daytime. I hobbled over to the surf and walked in the waves. It was probably the most serene place I have ever been.

With my foot still throbbing, I was finally able to doze off in my hut around four in the morning. At about nine I awoke drenched in sweat. I was so caught up in how drenched I was that I didn't notice how much better my foot felt. I guess my body had been able to fight off any potential infection. I sighed with relief and got up to change my wet clothes.

The following day, we boarded the boat that would take us back to mainland Panama to continue our migration north through Central America. That final day had thankfully had no other surprises. As we pulled away from the island we turned to go around a side of the island I hadn't seen yet. To my surprise, we could see from the boat that this side of the island was littered with trash. Lots of plastic, garbage bags, and various odds and ends that seemed out of place. I don't know where it came from, but it was such stark comparison to the pristine paradise on the other side. It seemed to fit into the theme of my time on San Blas, which was realizing how quickly situations can change. A few different times I went from relaxing vacation to panic in a matter of minutes. Looking back now, I realize that comparing a place like the San Blas Islands to the Western world is a perfect example of how rapidly human life has changed. Yet, even in a place like San Blas that seemed so far removed from the Western world, I could find things like Doritos and batteries, and the byproducts of the Western world were washing up on these previously untouched shores. Life for humans has gone through change on a much larger scale than what I saw comparing those islands to the Western world, and this change for humans has had greater consequences than an unpleasant shoreline.

Chapter 8: Humans in the Fast Lane

"Only recently have we come up with the technology to turn lazing around into a way of life. We've taken our sinewy, durable, hunter-gatherer bodies and plunked them into an artificial world of leisure."

– Christopher McDougall

In the grand scheme of things, life hasn't been around that long and human beings are barely a blip. The long history of multi-cellular life on Earth is important prerequisite information for understanding why humans are struggling with chronic disease. The timeline on the following page highlights some key points. Notice how all the action, as far as humans are concerned, has been packed into the very right side—so much so that I had to zoom in to the timeline twice.

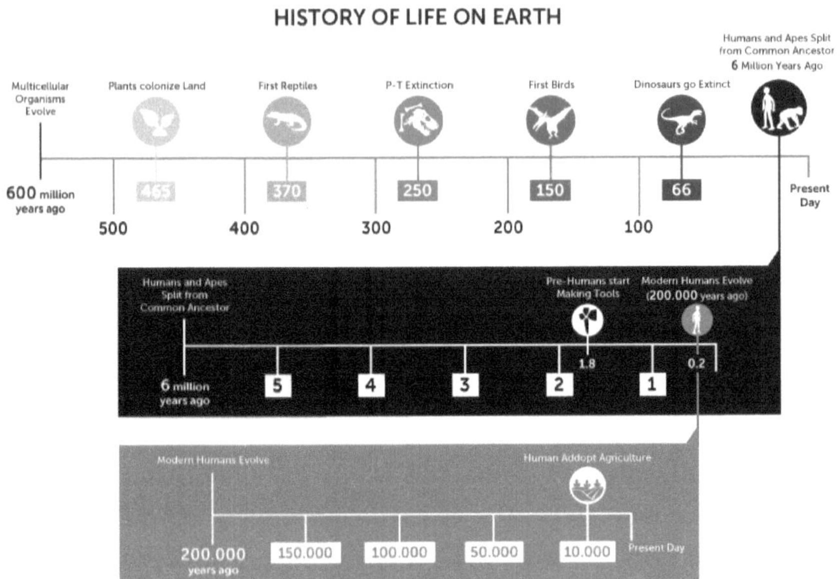

About 600 million years ago the first multi-cellular life formed on Earth. If we fast-forward through the evolution of plants, dinosaurs, the extinction of dinosaurs, and the evolution of first mammals, it brings us to about 6 million years ago when the first human-like ancestors branched off from our last common ancestor with apes. A lot more branching and dying off happened between then and 200,000-300,000 years ago when the first modern humans showed up. Compared to all of life on Earth, humans have not been here that long.

In his book, *A Brief History of Nearly Everything,* Bill Bryson puts it nicely by saying that if we were to put the entire existence of Earth (4,500 billion years or so) into the time span of a 24-hour day and look to see the amount of time that humans have been here, we would find that humans only appeared with 1 minute and 17 seconds left in that day. We are the new kids on the block. He also points out that if you were to put the length of one human's entire life in this 24-hour clock, it would be barely an instant of that day. Kind of makes you feel insignificant, doesn't it?

Aside from us not having been on Earth for very long, it is also important to step back and see what humans have been through since we arrived. The split that eventually lead to modern apes and modern humans happened about 6 million years ago. From then until modern humans emerged 200,000+ years ago we were nothing more than what we would think of as, well, apes. Then, from about 200,000+ years ago to about 40,000 years ago we were highly evolved apes, still nothing all that different from the other animals in the world. Then, for reasons that we are unsure of, this changed at that 40,000-year mark. This is referred to as the Great Leap Forward, and it happened in what is now Europe, where at the time Neanderthals were walking around. In *The Third Chimpanzee,* Jared Diamond tells us the significance of the Great Leap Forward:

> Until the Great Leap Forward, human culture had developed at a snail's pace for millions of years. That pace was dictated by the slow pace of genetic change. After the leap, cultural development no longer depended on genetic change. Despite negligible changes in our anatomy, there has been far more cultural evolution in the past forty thousand years than in the millions of years before.

The Great Leap Forward was just the beginning of the rapid advancement of the human species. As Diamond suggests, it was the evolutionary leap when our behavior and culture changed faster than our bodies could adapt. In this time people very similar to modern day people appeared and, according to archeological evidence, out-competed Neanderthals. Along with the appearance of these modern people came primitive tools, art, and trade. This Great Leap Forward was, relatively speaking, not that long ago. It was also just the first step toward massive changes in lifestyle that our ancestors would tumble through from then until now.

As important and sudden as the Great Leap Forward was for human beings, there were other quicker and more transformative changes to come. Arguably, the most significant of those major events took place about 10-12,000 years ago in what is now the Middle East and it changed the way humans ate, moved, and lived. That event is known as the Agricultural Revolution. The first archeological evidence of humans staying in one place and farming is seen during this time. Up until then all humans were hunter-gatherers moving around in small groups. It is important to realize that not all humans started farming all at once. In the beginning of the Agricultural Revolution there were still plenty of hunter-gatherers. However, this hunter-gatherer way of living declined as humans progressed. With the Agricultural Revolution the first humans began to show signs of the lifestyle that is by far the most common in the modern world.

We are not entirely sure why evolution drove humans to become farmers, but many have speculated. In *Why Nations Fail,* Daron Acemoglu and James A. Robinson suggest that, "The warming up of the climate was a huge critical juncture that formed the background of the Neolithic Revolution, where human societies made the transition to sedentary life, farming, and herding." Jared Diamond has suggested that this settling down happened where it did, the Middle East, because, at the time, there were many plants and animals in that area that were more susceptible to domestication than in other parts of the world. Could the combination of a warming planet, the right plants and animals in the right place at the right time, and the leaps in human evolutionary intellect have led to the tipping point that was the Agricultural Revolution? We may never know for sure.

Although the exact causes are unknown, what's important to realize is that the transition to farming was the single greatest change in the history of humans. It laid the foundation for more revolutions to come and had a monumental effect on our health. We can trace our epidemic of chronic disease back to the shift in lifestyle that occurred during this time. Unbeknownst to them, humans made a big trade-off when they gave up the hunter-gatherer lifestyle that they and their ancestors had thrived in for millions of years.

As in any trade-off, there were pros and cons. Arguing about whether the Agricultural Revolution had more benefits or drawbacks is irrelevant, but the cons shed light on the causes of our disease epidemic. Some of the benefits to this new way of life were being able to provide for ourselves while remaining in the same geographical location. This allowed humans to grow in numbers and spend more time developing and improving technology. In a short 9,000 years, we went from being a species of an estimated 5 million people with simplistic stone tools to 130 million with advanced civilizations like the Roman Empire. Technology would have been hard to transport in the nomadic hunter-gatherer lifestyle. But despite those pros this lifestyle change had many cons. For one, it made humans more dependent on crops, a food that would prove to be nutritionally inadequate compared to the wild foods humans had formerly eaten.

Evidence of this is found in the skeletal and dental comparisons of the Natufian people, some of the first farmers who lived from around 12,000 to 9,000 BC in what is now the Middle East. Prior to engaging in farming these people experienced optimal health. After they began farming they showed greater incidence of hypoplasia, a condition where malnutrition creates thin lines in peoples' tooth enamel. Early farmers seemed to have struggled while relying on crops.

Another example of the poor nutritional quality of food crops is provided by Jared Diamond in *The Third Chimpanzee*. He points out that corn first became domesticated in Central America thousands of years ago and became the staple of intensive farming around A.D. 1000. Archeologists found that once those societies switched to farming they experienced more cavities, anemia, tuberculosis, and osteoarthritis. Mortality rates increased for every age group as well. Archeologists have expressed to Diamond that before then, hunter-gatherer skeletons in that area were "so healthy it is somewhat discouraging to work with them." I guess that once an archeologist begins to study the skeletons of an ancient farmer in poor health, the pristine skeleton of a hunter-gather seems boring. Regardless, this is more evidence that relying on a select few crops compared to a very diverse wild food diet was not enough to meet the nutritional needs of a human being. And while modern farming practices have made crops more nutrient poor, the evidence that relying on crops had a negative effect on health has been there from the beginning. In the 1930s, Dr. Westin Price showed how dramatically health can be affected with abrupt dietary changes. We will talk more about Weston Price's work in Chapter 18.

Ailments resulting from reliance on low-quality food was just one health issue to arise with farming. This shift also allowed infectious disease to evolve and become a major cause of death. The close quarters of the Agricultural Revolution ushered in an era in which infectious diseases could readily pass from livestock to person and person to person. Prior to this, viruses and bacteria could not have survived long enough to find a new host. Humans and animals just weren't consistently that close to each other. Since viruses and bacteria reproduce at a fast rate, they were able to evolve and exploit our newfound proximity with great speed.

There is rarely only one cause to anything in our interconnected world, so living in close quarters may not be the sole explanation as to why infectious disease began to rise during this time. It has been known for a long time that healthy animal fats have potent anti-microbial properties.[1,2] Before we became reliant on crops, which had very few good fats, we were eating high animal fat diets that would have given us better protection against infectious disease. Some of these fats came with the meat we ate, but much of it was from us eating solely the fat of an animal. Building our bodies with these fats would have provided us protection from infection. You can imagine that the decrease in amounts of fat consumed by eating mainly crops left us vulnerable to the increase in infectious disease that potentially came from living in close quarters. But this is not the only effect that eating less fat had on humans. Many people don't realize that our brains used to be bigger than they are now—they have shrunk by 10% over the last 10,000 years.[3] This makes sense given that we are no longer eating enough of the quality high fat nutrients that largely make up our brain since shifting to crops as our main food source around 10,000 years ago. In her book, *Primal Fat Burner,* Nora Gedgaudas tells us that:

> Paleolithic hunters and gatherers derived around 90 percent of their caloric intake from the meat and fat of about one hundred to two hundred different species of wild animals. Small amounts of fibrous vegetables, greens, nuts, and fruits in season made up the rest. That is the natural diet of our species, and it was under these conditions that more than 99.99 percent of the human genome was forged.

She goes on to point out that since agriculture began "we have spent five hundred generations—less than 0.4 percent of our evolutionary history—eating a diet that is increasingly unnatural to our species."

Moving toward a life of agriculture also led to a class system, which created lack and surplus among the different classes. When living in small groups of hunter-gatherers, life was mostly spent trying to find food. As in most situations there were probably some individuals lower on the totem pole than others. This is even evident in one of our closest relatives, the chimpanzees. Anthropologist Craig Stanford has spent much of his career studying how the competition for meat leads to a hierarchy within groups of chimps. In his book, *The Hunting Apes,* he describes a scene where an alpha male is eating the meat of a monkey while "other members of the hunting party cluster around him attempting to get a morsel." He describes that younger, lower class chimps "sit on the forest floor below, hoping that fragments of bone or drops of blood fall to them." The alpha male ends up only sharing with select females—probably the mother of his children— and one other "longtime ally." I imagine it was very similar for early humans, and while chimps don't really have a class system, it shows how competition for food can create inequality.

Once agriculture was developed, humans started to live together in communities and civilizations where there was a little more looking out for each other than we see with the chimps. At the same time, whoever controlled the food had more power, just like the alpha male chimp. Food became the first currency, and with unequal access to it, a class system was born. It is interesting that much later in human history, types of food were still being used as currency. In Ancient Rome, armies required salt for soldiers, horses, and livestock, and at times soldiers were paid in salt. This is the origin of the word "salary" and explains the expression "worth his salt."

As with a class system and early currency, agriculture also brought about a need for government. Small groups of hunter-gatherers probably didn't have as many disagreements due to the fact that there just weren't as many opinions to go around. If there did happen to be a difference of opinions, those with opposing views could just go their separate ways. When life became sedentary, it became more difficult to pick up and leave. Therefore, people had to find better ways to resolve conflicts over land and commodities, which lead to early governing bodies and politics. Sometimes I feel that politicians are just as ineffective today as they would be if we stuck a modern politician in with the first farmers.

Another interesting interpretation of the cause for the Agricultural Revolution comes to light when taking into account that in some parts of the world, we have found archeological evidence that suggests that human organization, such as politics and religion, formed quite a while before farming. This suggests that at some point evolution favored humans with cooperative and social tendencies, which enabled them to organize themselves into societies, even without the presence of domesticated plants and animals. This interpretation proposes that humans formed larger groups, and farming was the solution to keeping larger populations fed, rather than farming allowing us to form large groups and stay in one place.

This is quite possible considering that part of the 1.4% difference in genes between us and chimps includes our ability to communicate at a high level and work together more efficiently. Perhaps those plants and animals that were adaptable to human needs got a large evolutionary boost as we began altering the environment. Whatever the sequence of events, farming—the Agriculture Revolution—was a huge change to the lifestyle that humans—or any life on Earth—had known for millions of years before. Up until the Agricultural Revolution we were at the mercy of the environment to push our slow evolution. Suddenly humans became the fittest animal around, not because we fit well in the environment, but because we manipulated our environment to suit us.

With agriculture, we began to "domestically select" many life forms around us, un-syncing them and ourselves from the innate wisdom of natural selection. This allowed us to multiply and eventually become the dominant species on Earth. However, plants like wheat, corn, and rice, along with animals like cows, pigs, and sheep, are right below us in number. The more copies of a species' genes on the planet, the more likely the species is to survive. Given that there are over 7 billion humans alive today, I'd say we're covered in that department, but so are the domesticated plants and animals we have brought with us. As successful as this may sound for us and these species, I believe the Agricultural Revolution was a bad move for both. We are very dependent on our domesticated species and they are dependent on us. If we lost them a large part of our population would be lost due to food shortage, and if they lost us they would lose large portions of their populations because we wouldn't be around to keep them alive and reproducing in the ways we have for 10,000 years. This is a delicate dependency.

Out in the harshness of the wild, small groups of humans needed to be ready for anything that was thrown at them, like predators, tough winters, or food scarcity. Their diets had to be spot on to ensure survival through these harsh times. Once humans started farming they were able to grow their numbers, ensure a source of food, and lessen their vulnerabilities by living indoors. Despite these things, when studying the Agricultural Revolution, I think we make the false assumption that it resulted in an easier life. It may have been nice to stay in one spot, multiply in numbers, and be sheltered from dangers, but large sacrifices were made.

The Bible is enlightening to read through this lens. In Genesis, Chapter 3, God punishes Adam and Eve for partaking in the forbidden fruit. His punishment for Adam was that he would no longer be able to eat freely from the Garden of Eden (aka nature) saying, "Cursed is the ground because of you! In toil you shall eat its yield all the days of your life. Thorns and thistles shall it bear for you, and you shall eat the grass of the field. By the sweat of your brow you shall eat bread." As for Eve, God said, "I will intensify your toil in childbearing; in pain you shall bring forth children." Given that the Bible has been interpreted in many ways and is still open for interpretation, I read these verses as aligning with the arguments of this chapter. We have discussed how the backbreaking work of this new farming life may have created harder lives for humans than they previously lived. Archeological evidence also shows that the human pelvis became narrower after adopting agriculture, which given the large size of our brain, would have made childbirth more difficult and painful. Perhaps whoever wrote the book of Genesis was merely describing some of the effects of man coming out of nature and beginning to rely on farming for food. It is entirely possible that the author attributed the detrimental effects as punishment from their god. Remember when we discussed how an ancient people suffering with chronic disease would have determined that their gods had turned on them? Perhaps whoever wrote this part of the Bible thought the exact same thing.

I hope that by now I have convinced you that the Agricultural Revolution had a detrimental effect on the health of humans, or at least sparked your curiosity. Let's keep moving on down the line from the Agricultural Revolution toward modern day. After the onset of the Agricultural Revolution, we see the rise and fall of many great civilizations, such as Mesopotamia, Ancient Egypt, the Roman Empire, and the Mayan Empire. Humans kept trucking along in these civilizations, eating, praying, and fighting for the better part of the last 10,000 years, until more Revolution-scale changes happened in rapid succession. The Scientific and Industrial revolutions each happened within the last 500 years and also contributed to our health crisis.

I truly believe that humans were oblivious to what harm they were doing to themselves during the Agricultural Revolution. How could they have analyzed the risk/benefit trade off? However, in the Scientific and Industrial Revolutions, I think that we humans finally got too smart for our own good. I say this because we started doing anything and everything to advance society. We started doing things just because we could, and sometimes I wonder if anyone stopped to think if we should do them, or at least how they may affect us. To be fair, evolution didn't enter scientific knowledge until the mid-1800s, which was after those revolutions, and as we discussed before, infection hid many of the effects of these revolutions by killing us before the symptoms of these changes could appear.

Some of the greatest advancements and thinkers in human history came out of these two revolutions. The innovation of those times propelled us to what I think is the best time to ever be alive and human. However, when trying to trace the roots of our health crisis of today these revolutions end up being major contributors. The technology that came out of these revolutions ultimately lead to the unnecessary processing of our food, the introduction of many toxic chemicals into our bodies, the shift toward a stressful capitalist society that places the value of money over anything else, and the changing of our deeply ingrained movement habits. So much has changed in the past 500 years, and things are still changing so fast that none of us can really keep up, myself included. The newest smartphone will probably become available and then become outdated before I finish writing this chapter.

Let's go through some of the major changes we have seen as a result of these revolutions. When out in the wild, humans ate many different types of nutrient rich foods. Since the Agricultural Revolution we started eating less variety, and since the Industrial Revolution we have limited that variety even more. Today, three nutritionally poor crops—wheat, rice, and corn—account for the majority of calories consumed by humans. We eat most of those calories in the form of highly processed versions of those crops, which are even more nutritionally poor. We also feed the majority of our livestock these foods, making the meat we get from them also nutritionally poor. Limiting the amount and sources of nutrients has not turned out well for us.

The Industrial Revolution also contributed to poor health by allowing us to access food beyond what we can grow, forage, or hunt in our local geographical region. It became possible to easily ship massive amounts of food from all over the world to places, and people, that were not used to having those foods. If you are the product of humans who lived in northern Europe, your genes come from people who ate cows, milk, cold weather vegetables, fish, oats, and berries. At the drop of a hat these peoples had access to tropical fruit and fish. You have to think their bodies would be a little confused at the arrival of an avocado or coconut and may not accept those foods readily. So much attention is being paid to this idea that one day we may be able to test peoples' genes and tell them exactly what to eat based on their ancestors' diets.

The third major change we have seen since the Scientific and Industrial Revolutions also pertains to our food. In this case it is the amount of toxicants we consume. In *Food Forensics,* Mike Adams gives us some statistics about recent chemical use on those three crops (plus soy) that make up the majority of the American diet. He says:

Global pesticide use has continued to increase since the second half of the twentieth century, with more than 5.2 billion pounds of herbicides, insecticides, and fungicides in use as of 2007, and global sales headed toward an estimated $57 billion by 2016. According to Food & Water Watch, herbicide use has increased by 26 percent in the United States just since 2001.

The amount of chemicals our bodies come in contact with on a daily basis is increasing rapidly, and our food is only one way that we are getting exposed. According to Herbert Needleman, who spent his life studying the effect of chemicals on children, at least 70,000 new chemical compounds have been invented and dispersed into our environment since 1950, and only a fraction of these have been tested for human toxicity. We are, by default, conducting a massive clinical toxicology trial, and our children and grandchildren are the experimental animals. That's pretty scary, but it doesn't stop there.

Heavy metals like lead, mercury, cadmium, arsenic, and aluminum became abundant in our environment during the Industrial Revolution. These elements were deposited deep in the earth's crust billions of years ago, which means that life evolved without them—up until we found uses for them and started digging them up. Our physiologies have no need and no place for these elemental metals. We have all heard of fish being toxic because of the bioaccumulation of mercury. Fish store mercury because they have no use for it and no way to get rid of it. Fortunately, we can get rid of them but not without great effort by our bodies. When ingested, these metals wreak havoc on the mitochondria present in every cell, which are essential for our ability to make energy. Also, due to the fact that these metals are new to the scene, our bodies are not as effective at getting them out as they are with other kinds of toxins. Therefore, many of the metals we come in contact with end up being stored in tissues, including in our brains. Our exposure to toxic metals is also a growing problem.

Another danger relatively new to the scene is genetically modified organisms (GMOs). GMOs are plants that have had their genes bioengineered for certain traits, and they are out of control. According to GMO Compass, the global hectares of GMOs grew from 1.7 million in 1996 to nearly 140 million hectares in 2009. Everyday people are eating food with genetic information that has been instantly changed by human intervention. Let's think about that. This book makes the argument that humans are having trouble with the changes that have happened in the last 10,000 years through agriculture practices, so what makes us think that we will be able to handle a direct genetic change that happens effectively overnight? What happens when we eat a combination of genetic information that our bodies have never seen before? What happens when our children eat it for their entire lives? No one is exactly sure.

The Scientific and Industrial Revolutions also yielded the capitalist society we live in today. Within capitalism, we only have to be good at one thing—our job—which allows us to make money. Everything else can be outsourced by using that money. This creates a society of people that will do anything and everything to attain money, because what we need to survive can (and many times must) be acquired with it. If we don't make money, or suddenly lose all our money, then our chances of survival drop dramatically. Every time I see a homeless person I am reminded that our society is so dependent on money that its absence threatens our very lives. Conversely, when we lived in the wild, a great many sources could provide us with sustenance, shelter, and all the necessities of survival. Relying on a single source for survival makes for a very fragile and stressful environment. If you were to ask most people the top three sources of stress, money would be there for almost everyone.

Pre-agricultural peoples had stress too, but only in situations where stressful responses were needed to stay alive, like being chased by a predator. Since our day-to-day survival is dependent on money, we spend a large majority of our time fearing for the health and well-being of ourselves and our families because of not having enough of it. Having constant life-threatening stress responses to non-life-threatening situations was not the dominant way of life over the millions of years that humans were evolving in the wild. Our biology is not set up for that.

Our mental well-being does not escape the effects of our change in lifestyle. Depression and other mental illnesses are chronic diseases as well. In his 2012 research article entitled *Depression is a Disease of Modernity: Explanations for Increasing Prevalence*, Brandon H. Hidaka uses this reasoning to explain the increase in depression saying:

> The growing burden of chronic diseases, which arise from an evolutionary mismatch between past human environments and modern day living, may be central to rising rates of depression. Declining social capital and greater inequality and loneliness are candidate mediators of a depressogenic social milieu. Modern populations are increasingly overfed, malnourished, sedentary, sunlight-deficient, sleep-deprived, and socially isolated. These changes in lifestyle each contribute to poor physical health and affect the incidence and treatment of depression.

Our activity levels and types have also dramatically changed since the Agricultural Revolution and even further during the Scientific and Industrial Revolutions. About 10,000 years ago we quickly went from being constantly on the move (hunting for food and water), to living in one spot doing the backbreaking work of farming. Then, over the last 200 years, we invented machines to do our work for us, which allowed us to transition to doing a lot of sitting. Scientists have compared the bones of modern day people to the fossilized remains of hunter-gatherer people and have found that the shapes of our bones are formed structurally weaker and our trabecular bone—the inner, honey-comb-like layer of bone—is less dense.[4] The type and amount of movements that we do as we grow affects how our bones form. The way hunter-gatherers lived resulted in well-formed bones of superior strength compared to our own.

To help illustrate one last way that our lifestyle affects us and the planet, think about how we once were completely occupied by attaining what was necessary (food, water, shelter) to keep us alive long enough to pass on genes. It would have taken up the majority of our time on Earth. In today's society those things come easily for most. We work 40 hours a week to make money so that we can easily buy the things that keep us alive. We have created a lot of free time for ourselves, which has resulted in the many forms of entertainment we have available to us today. The readily available essentials in today's world make our lives so boring and monotonous that we need endless forms of entertainment to occupy the excess time we have created. This quest to be entertained has had a major negative impact on our planet. I am not saying that you should feel bad about going to the movies, but just stop and think about how often you do things to entertain yourself and how much it costs (money, resources) to bring that entertainment to you. Think about what other living things in the world, including other humans, may have had to go through in order for you to have what you need to be entertained. Maybe there are ways to entertain yourself that will also create a healthier you and a healthier world. We will discuss this more in Chapter 16.

Okay, so we've drastically changed the way we live over the last 10,000 years—that's still a long time, right? Maybe 10,000 years since our first major lifestyle change doesn't seem like a short time, but remember the timeline introduced at the beginning of this chapter. For 600 million years life evolved sustaining itself in the natural environment, for 6 million years our human ancestors evolved in that same environment, and for 200,000 years modern humans evolved in that same environment. Then 40,000 years ago we had a Great Leap Forward that eventually propelled us to our first drastic change in lifestyle at about 10,000 years ago. You can see that these pivotal changes keep happening with less and less time separating them. The rate of change hasn't stopped increasing since it started. Relatively speaking, humankind's lifestyle upheavals happened rapidly and recently. Remember, though, that the evolutionary process is and will remain slow. A fast environmental change paired with a slow evolutionary response has consequences.

Jared Diamond says it well in The *Third Chimpanzee*: "Hunter-gatherers practiced the most successful and long-persistent lifestyle in the career of our species. In contrast we are still struggling with the problems into which we descended with agriculture, and it is unclear whether we can solve them." He writes that if the history of humanity is a 24-hour clock, "we lived as hunter-gatherers for nearly the whole of that day, from midnight through dawn, noon, and sunset." We don't get agriculture until 11:54 P.M.

I hope by now you see what I am getting at. The reason for our decline in health is the accelerated change in our daily environment and lifestyle to something nearly unrecognizable when compared to how our environment shaped us for millions of years. We do not reproduce fast enough for evolution to make us resilient to our man-altered environments, and we are witnessing the repercussions in the form of our health epidemic.

To be clear, I am saying that the chronic disease epidemic we are facing is a direct result of the human way of life changing so quickly that the slow process of evolution has not allowed us to adapt to it. The symptoms and diseases we experience are the body responding to being in an environment it is not fit for. It is similar to when we see wild animals struggling to thrive in a zoo.

Compared to the duration all life has been on Earth, our time here is pretty insignificant, and the time that we have been farming and enjoying the advancements of the Scientific and Industrial Revolutions even less so. In the corporation of earth, modern humans are the fresh-out-of-college, super-smart new employee. However, instead of sitting back and learning from the employees that have been at the company much longer than us and then using our smarts to improve on what was already there, we quickly rose to CEO and did whatever we wanted without weighing the consequences. We changed the company so that it best suited us, and now we have threatened to take the whole company down. Others in the company may be suffering more than we are right now, but our chronic disease epidemic is proof that we are not immune to our own manipulations. If the company goes down, we go down with it.

Chapter 9: Finding My Niche in Portlandia

I spent four years in Portland, Oregon training to be a chiropractor. Much of my time in the latter half of that training was in a treatment room as an intern, gaining experience in patient care. Many of my early patients left lasting impressions on me. They include a 96-year-old man who never seemed to remember that I was his doctor and my first pregnant patient, who happened to be a best friend's wife. I felt great responsibility for these patients. There were also a few that really threw me for a loop.

One day I was sitting in a treatment room at our school's downtown clinic, which was designed to give care to under-privileged and homeless people. We interns had recently been deemed ready to see patients under the supervision of an attending, but without the attending having to be in the room. We were encouraged to team up and treat patients together. In this instance, my friend Kevin was the primary intern, and I was the secondary, scribing for him as he did an exam.

Marlene sat on the table. She was a handful. She was a homeless woman in her mid-40s and from the moment she came into the clinic she was letting everyone know how excited she was to see a chiropractor. She had a very pleasant face that you could tell had seen rough times. She was very positive and nice but also very loud and not afraid to be noticed. Our attending gave us the signal to hurry up and get her in a room, though I'm sure everyone in the clinic could hear her no matter where she was in the clinic.

Once we got in the room she got super excited and said, "There it is, there's my chiropractic table!" She starting asking us what position we wanted her in first. "Want me to lay face down?" she said, and then she lay face down. "How 'bout on my side?" and then she lay on her side. "Nah, I bet you want me to sit first?" She sat right up. After we took her history, we eventually got her into the flow of an exam. Many of the tests were negative, and I got the sense that she feared we weren't going to treat her if we couldn't find anything wrong with her. She started doing something strange.

She was lying on her back and we asked her to bend her leg and put it on the table, and she said that all of the sudden she couldn't bend her right knee, even though she had already bent it many times. She looked at Kevin and said, "You're going to have to bend it for me." From that point on she would not move her right knee in any way unless Kevin moved it for her. When we asked her to lie face down, her lower leg remained bent at the knee sticking straight off the table. Kevin went over and straightened her leg until it rested on the table. When we asked her to sit up she sat straight up, but her right leg remained straight, jutting out from the table. Kevin went over and bent it to a normal sitting position. "Thank you," she said in a way that you would if someone held a door open for you.

We asked her if she had ever had any knee pain or if this had ever happened before. She said that it was not painful and that five minutes ago during the exam was the first time it had ever happened to her. "Isn't that weird? I must be really messed up," she said. When we told her that we were going to treat her, she said, "Oh, thank goodness. I don't know how much longer I can live like this!" After treatment we told her that we wanted to see her next week and that she should schedule with the front desk. As she was walking out of the room (bending her knee just fine, I might add) she turned and looked straight at me and said, "You look just like Tom Cruise." Then she turned to Kevin and said, "And you look just like Brad Pitt!" in a surprised sort of way as if she had just realized this. She walked straight to the front desk and requested to make an appointment with Tom Cruise and Brad Pitt for the same time next week. Suddenly our receptionists had nicknames to tease us with.

While many people might find it hard to be envious of someone like Marlene, it was hard not to be inspired by her positive attitude. Inspiration is not something that most people in Portland feel when it comes to the homeless, though. When having conversations with people about living in Portland, mention of the amount of homeless people will come up more often than not. People who love Portland will often cite it as one of the very few negative things about the city, and people who hate Portland just have another reason to hate it. I saw homeless people a lot while using the excellent public transportation system for which Portland is known. Now I find it strange that homelessness is even a thing at all, even though it seems "normal" because we have become so accustomed to it in our society.

Humans require food and water to survive. To thrive they need a little more than that, like emotional connection, light, contact with nature, etc. Humans lived for thousands of years before civilization required money for survival; now we have created a society so dependent on that one thing that if you don't have enough you find yourself in a dire situation. Civilization is our attempt to control our environments in order to make our lives easier and less susceptible to the relentlessness of natural selection. In doing this we have created many symptoms of civilization, homeless populations being one of them.

As much as civilization has tried to control its environment for the sake of making human life easier, Portland is one example of a culture within our society that has taken things very far. I really enjoyed my time in Portland but didn't realize how different a place it was until I left. There are obviously many different walks of human life in Portland, but it is well known for being a haven for hippies, environmentalists, vegans, bike commuters, natural healers, outdoor enthusiasts, artists, and microbrewers. I was no exception. I spent four years there and despite only having a car for a few months of this time, I found it quite easy to get where I needed to go via Portland's abundant bike lanes and public transportation. I also decided to become vegan (not my best decision) while I was there and my social life didn't suffer in the slightest because nearly every restaurant in town had vegan options and even had vegan beer, so I could go out with friends and still eat. People also love chiropractors in Portland. There was one on every corner, and they were all in business. I got very positive responses when I told people that I was training to become a chiropractor. Portland is so health conscious that they even voted to keep fluoride (a proven neuro toxin) out of their drinking water, so I didn't even have to worry about filtering it out.

If you are into these types of things, Portland makes it very easy to do them and not catch much flak from anyone who disagrees with your lifestyle. Portland caters to the lifestyle that a majority of its inhabitants love. Much like humans created civilization in the attempts to dodge the struggle of survival of the fittest out in the wild, Portlanders enjoy their lifestyle with ease. You can imagine how much more difficult it is to live this way in other parts of the country, like the rural southeastern United States for instance.

This is one thing I thought about a lot when I left Portland. I knew how hard it would be to continue the lifestyle once I left. I had no idea, however, that I would later come to realize that there are major consequences to a species being smart enough to control their environment in such a major way.

Chapter 10: Masters of Niche Construction

"By changing the physical world to fit his requirements—or wishes—man has almost done away with the need for biological adaptation on his part. He has thus established a biological precedent and is tempting fate, for biological fitness achieved through evolutionary adaptation has been so far the most dependable touchstone of permanent success in the living world."

— Rene Dubos

Now that you can see how quickly and dramatically our way of life has changed since the Agricultural Revolution, let's delve deeper into our incredible relationship to the environment. I'm not talking about polluted oceans, disappearing rainforests, and climate change necessarily (though those are also important) but more about our personal environments—the stimuli that our bodies come in contact with or experience every day. Remember from Chapter 6 that, per *Principles of Evolutionary Medicine,* the environment of an organism is defined as "the sum of all the external conditions and stimuli that it experiences, including climate, nutrient supply, social structure resulting from other members of its own species, and threats from other species in the form of predation, parasitism, or infection." So for us this would include the food you eat, the water you bathe in, the products you use, the chemicals you come in contact with, the air you breathe, the stress you experience, etc. From here on out when I refer to our personal environments this is the environment I am referring to.

When it comes to determining what creates health or causes disease I am not only concerned with the environment your body encounters today, but the culmination of everything that you have ever come in contact with or has happened to you throughout your lifetime. For example, right from the start, were you a natural birth or C-section? It matters, and, depending on which one it was, it is one of the first stimuli that can have a positive or negative effect on your health. I could then ask if you were breastfed or formula fed. It also matters. Before you are even a day old there are two opportunities to either create an environment for health or create an environment for disease. But why do these variations in our personal environments matter? I mean, we're still here, aren't we? We are still growing as a species, so who cares if our personal environments have changed. Well, when you start to investigate the trends of chronic disease you many come to some eye-opening realizations.

The leading diseases of our modern world (heart disease, cancer, diabetes) are not old diseases. They are new, having showed up only around 10,000 years ago and developed into major problems only over the last 100–200 years or so.[1] In fact, no matter what chronic ailment or disease plagues us, I believe that it can probably be traced back to the changes in our way of life that started with the Agricultural Revolution. It is hard to ignore the timely correlation between dramatic changes in our way of life, archeological evidence of weaker bodies, and the eventual rise in chronic disease. I think it is safe to say these changes play a major role—if not the only role—in our current health struggles.

From my initial interest in health to when I began to grasp the causes of rising chronic disease, I went through a lot of trial and error. Then, I finally framed my journey with the right questions. How do animals evolve? What pressures induce that evolution? How do humans fit in with the natural world? What has changed for humans? Once I found the right questions the answers were revealing and exciting. You can't change the environment or a species too fast without throwing off the equilibrium.

In the geologic record there is evidence of five mass extinctions that have happened on Earth at various times. They are thought to be the result of natural catastrophic events. You know, a giant meteor strikes Earth and causes very drastic and timely changes in the earth's environment or maybe the earth's volcanoes have a volcano party all at once—things like that. Things living at the time of one of these events couldn't possibly evolve quickly enough to fit their changing environments and therefore became extinct. Fortunately, the recent changes in our personal environment are happening slowly enough that they are not killing us. However, they are happening fast enough to have negative effects on our health. It has happened in such a way that we can't clearly point a finger as to why our health is declining. The dinosaurs didn't need to gather around a table and discuss what started their extinction or spend trillions of dollars combating the effects of their catastrophic event. It was pretty obvious. For us, there haven't been any jump-out-in-front-of-your-face obvious events that lead to our situation. Because of this, society is stuck in the middle of this growing disease epidemic where millions of people are struggling through life and floating from doctor to doctor looking for answers.

Concern grows when you dig a little deeper and look at what's been happening on a genetic level since the Agricultural Revolution. For millions of years evolution selected the best genes to pass to the next generation, but after all that has happened to humans in the recent past we may be creating weaker human genes with each new generation. To understand this we first need to learn a little about a shift in genetic thinking that has happened in the last 20 years. When it comes to the role our genes play in determining the person that we are, it turns out not all our genes are set in stone and most of them can be influenced to act one way or another. The science of epigenetics has revolutionized the way we think about genes and the diseases they "cause."

I want you to think about diseases as being in one of two categories. Those categories are Mendelian (as in Gregor Mendel, the discoverer of inheritable traits) and multifactorial diseases. Mendelian diseases are diseases where a single mutation in a gene is directly inherited, having one cause. Examples of these are diseases like cystic fibrosis and sickle cell anemia. Multifactorial diseases are those that are caused by a number of different factors, and the individual's risk of getting them is determined by the combination of weak influence from many different genes and strong influence of developmental and environmental factors. These are our very common diseases like heart disease, asthma, and cancer. To be clear, there is no single gene that is the cause of any multifactorial disease, and researching for a gene that causes them is a waste of time. Epigenetics gives us all the answers we need when it comes to the cause of these diseases.

The basic premise of epigenetics is that our genes do not determine the outcome of our health as the Western medical model would have us think. Genes are much like the hard drive of a computer. Once it is built there isn't much you can change about it unless you open it up and do hard drive surgery. Our immediate environment tells our hard drive (or genes) how to operate. I liken this to software. Software tells our hard drive to run a certain operating system, web browser, or screen saver. The software (our environment) can change and be changed, and the hard drive (our genes) cannot be changed but is substantially influenced by the software. In functional medicine circles the saying goes, 'Your genes load the gun, but you environment pulls the trigger.'

In Petri dishes, developmental biologist Bruce Lipton proved that you can change the functionality of cells by altering the environment in the dish. He showed that the genes in the cells did not predetermine how the cell worked but that the cell performed tasks based on what environmental stimuli were present around it.[2] This proved that our cells were not preprogrammed by the genetic code they contained. The genes received signals from their outside world that told them what to do. Thanks to this experiment, and Lipton's further work, we now know that our genes are not rigid codes with one outcome, but have many outcomes that can result from following different instructions. Gene expression is based largely on how we instruct them, and our instruction is the way we choose to live our lives.

We may be able to influence the genes we are born with but it's important to recognize that we can't entirely change them. We have all heard of people who smoke, drink, and eat a terrible diet their whole lives yet they live to be 100 years old with very few health issues. We also have all heard of those instances when a child has cancer. This can be explained by genetic variation. Some families have genes that happen to be fit for dealing with the drastic environmental changes that have created the world we live in. Their reckless lifestyles don't seem to affect their health or lifespan too much. Others have genes that are not fit to deal with this environment and they end up with illness earlier in life. I refer to this concept as the "hardiness of genes." People with hardy genes can be more reckless, and people with less hardy genes have to work harder to be free of disease. You can look at your family health history to get a general idea of how hardy your genes are; just remember that our environments are changing ever faster and people today are being exposed to things that the genes of their parents and grandparents never had to confront. You have to work with the genes you are given, but regardless of the genes you have, you can influence and instruct them so that they express a healthier version of you. Most of us probably are somewhere in between having hardy and weak genes. The point is that there is nothing we can do about the hand we were dealt, but health is created when the right combination of genes and environment are present and so we have more control than we might think.

This is huge! If you have a chronic disease it is because your personal environment has been telling your genes to react in a way that modern medicine would classify as a disease. Therefore, if you can change your personal environment to instruct your genes differently, you'll get a better health outcome. We will talk more about strategies to do this in Part Three.

As good as it is that we can influence our genes, it does have a big downside. We've had a quick and substantial change in our human way of life, and we have genetic expression of genes that we know are influenced by that altered way of life. That is a cause for concern, especially if you look at the instructions our environments have been giving our genes since the Agricultural Revolution.

If we give our genes the instructions to cause illness, like we have been doing for a while now, then those genes are in a weakened state. Okay, you may be thinking, so we just fix our personal environment and everything is better—right? Unfortunately, the truth of the matter is more complicated. If our genes are in that weakened state when we have a child, then some of that weaker gene state gets inherited. Not only are we out of sync with our natural evolution, we are defying it by selecting the weaker genes to pass on. On the flip side, if we really take care of ourselves before having a child, those awesome genes get passed on. Which genes do you want to give your kids?

One of the major stimuli that can cause a weaker gene state is those heavy metals we talked about earlier. In *Food Forensics*, Mike Adams discusses the harmful effects heavy metals have on genes across generations:

> Epigenetic inheritance of toxic side effects from dietary exposure to heavy metals means that toxicity is trans-generational. This means that the toxic environment in which we live today will negatively impact future generations for an unknown number of generations, even if we eliminate all exposure starting tomorrow.

And it's not just heavy metals that can have this effect. Our current lifestyles tend to expose us to many things that create weaker genes. I would conjecture that this genetic inheritance of weaker and weaker genes started when humans adapted an agricultural lifestyle and starting living more sedentary lives. Those with the absolute weakest genes for that environment probably didn't make it and their weak genes died with them. Despite having weaker genes, those who did make it continued to pass on those genes generation after generation, until modern day. Every time humans experienced another change in personal environment without having time to evolve to it, our genetic pool probably got a little bit weaker. If dealing with the unnatural environment wasn't enough for our bodies to handle, we must also try to combat it armed with weakened genes. Let's not be too negative though. If you look at this positively you will see that if we can influence them to be weaker, then we can influence them to go in the opposite direction as well. It may take time, but through conscientious decisions I'll lay out in Part Three, there is opportunity to reverse the situation we have made for ourselves.

There is another angle to this argument that our genes are becoming less fit for the environment in which we live. Stephen Jay Gould and Niles Eldridge have coined the term "punctuated equilibrium." In a nutshell, punctuated equilibrium describes the phenomenon that a secluded group of a given species will evolve faster because small variations in traits have greater impacts on smaller populations just because there are fewer sets of genes to change. You find this sort of thing in geographically secluded places like islands, as Darwin probably did in the Galapagos Islands. This principle leads me to ask, if smaller secluded groups of a species evolve faster, then do large, non-secluded species evolve slower? What happens when a species, like humans, becomes so numerous and so globally intertwined that it's almost impossible to find secluded populations where slight genetic variation can result in faster evolution of better traits? Are we headed in a direction that makes punctuated equilibrium impossible? Is being so over-populated slowing our ability to evolve in the changing world?

Let's take a closer look at the way we are becoming a globally intertwined species—effectively outsourcing the Western way of life across the globe—and how that has consequences. There used to be many cultures with their own cuisines, but now many cultures are adopting an unhealthy Standard American Diet (aptly abbreviated "SAD"). Now that the agribusiness and food corporations that drive the Standard American Diet seem to be unlimited in where they can supply food, more and more of the world is adopting aspects of that diet. From a health perspective, no group of people, no matter the race or ethnicity, does well on this diet. Curiously, however, it seems that those of European descent have less incidence of chronic disease than do those of non-European descent on the SAD. I will let Jared Diamond help me theorize as to why this might be with a passage from his book, *The World Until Yesterday*. Using the Nauruan people who live in the Pacific Islands as an example, he discusses how Europeans may be hardier against the Standard American Diet because dietary changes occurred sooner for them, before the pace of change hit breakneck speed.

He proposes that Europeans may have lived through an epidemic of diabetes brought on by a slow but steady increase in food availability occurring between the 1400s and 1700s. Over the course of those centuries, more gene hardy individuals would have survived and those weaker died off "as a result of many infants of diabetic mothers dying at birth, diabetic adults dying younger than other adults, and children and grandchildren of those diabetic adults dying of neglect or reduced material support," he says. The result is a population of individuals with diabetes-resistant genes. By contrast, in modern epidemics:

> Abundant and continually reliable food arrived *suddenly* [my emphasis]—within a decade for Nauruans, and within just a month for Yemenite Jews. The results were sharply peaked surges in diabetes's prevalence to 20-50% that have been occurring right under the eyes of modern diabetologists. Those increases will probably wane quickly (as already observed among Nauruans), as individuals with a thrifty genotype become eliminated by natural selection within a mere generation or two. [....] In effect, Pimas, Nauruans, Wanigelas, educated urban Indians, and citizens of wealthy oil-producing Arab nations are telescoping into a single generation the lifestyle changes and consequent rise and fall of diabetes

that unfolded over the course of many centuries in Europe.

Not only does this show that quick changes in diet have an impact on human health, as was seen during the Agricultural Revolution, but it also shows that since we now have "diabetologists," those populations like the Nauruans are not evolving away from diabetes because modern medicine can keep them alive to pass on their genes, whereas in Europe 300-600 years ago they would have died before passing on their genes. Although of course we absolutely want to prevent populations from dying from diabetes, it illustrates how we are out of sync with one of the basic mechanisms of evolution that is meant to keep us fit.

The global effect of the Standard American Diet is causing us to lose genetic diversity and genetic diversity is essential for the survival of a species. For millions of years evolution operated in such a way that it created strong genes that were best adapted to the environment. Those genes of humans that were less fit for the wild environment died off leaving only the more fit genes to contribute to the gene pool. After millions of years we were evolved to thrive in that wild environment. I am reminded how well adapted humans must have been before 10,000 years ago when I watch nature shows. I marvel at all the amazing feats that living things in nature can do. They are such masters of their environments. I bet humans were like that, too. Then, about 10,000 years ago, that strong set of genes slowly started to unravel. As we have gradually become a global society, we are dragging those humans with stronger, wilder genes, like the Nauruans, down to the level of weak westerner genes.

So I guess you can say we are devolving? Think about it—if natural evolution tends to create genes fit for the environment they are in, and we are creating weaker and weaker genes that are not a great fit for our modern environment, then technically, we are devolving. What's more, we are defying the fact that in nature those individuals with the least fit genes would be less likely to pass on their genes because they would die or not have the opportunity to mate. In today's society those of us with chronic diseases have genes that are not fit for the treacherous environment we have created, yet we still have a high chance of passing on those unfit genes.

Personally, I am a perfect example of how our technological advancements give us protection from the natural selection processes that we otherwise wouldn't stand a chance against! My own genes had a terrible response to the modern environment that we live in today. All the inflammatory conditions I had as a child were consequences of my body taking that environmental instruction and creating a bad expression of the genes I have. At 9 years old, when I was diagnosed with type 1 diabetes, that should have been it for me. I should have died sometime soon after that, and my unfit genes would have gone with me. Yet here I am. By humans learning to extract insulin from animals and then eventually learning to make synthetic insulin, I am still here. I can still pass on my unfit genes and therefore contribute to the devolving of our species. It is similar with type 2 diabetes as well— through the use of insulin and diabetic drugs we are not reversing type 2 diabetes to create stronger genes in those people, which is relatively simple to do through lifestyle modification; we are just allowing those with diabetes to pass on the tendency to get the disease to their children. Looking at it through this lens it seems that Western medicine's approach to diabetes is unintentionally increasing its prevalence in our society.

Through modern advances in technology, we have made it so that when someone is born with a genetic mutation that makes them less fit for our modern environment, it is very likely that we can keep them alive, and they will be able to pass on their genes. This is creating weaker genes for our species as a whole, and it also takes away any advantage that those born with an advantageous mutation would have. Remember, from Chapter 5, the random genetic mutations that can give certain individuals an advantage for survival? It is these advantageous mutations that create characteristics among species that help to push our species forward and allow us to survive in an ever-changing environment.

When the environment changes as rapidly as it has for us in the last 10,000 years, a species can either evolve (given enough time), it can migrate, or it can create more stable conditions by way of what is called niche construction. Some examples of this are the temperature-controlled mounds we see built by termites or the river-influencing dams built by beavers. We have taken niche construction to a whole new level, and one consequence of being the ultimate niche constructors, creating conditions where it is easy for everyone to survive and pass on their genes, is that we are essentially neutralizing mutations and evolutionary advantages that would help us survive the quicker and quicker changes we experience.

Our massive niche construction has in a way made us weaker. Many diehard evolutioners say that if we were intelligently designed, then why do so many of us need protection from the sun's rays, need eyeglasses, or need knee replacements? Well, while I agree a creator might want to make their creation more durable in their environment, there is more at play here. I don't think we would be so vulnerable to the natural world if we hadn't torn ourselves away, at such a quick pace, from the environment we evolved in for millions of years. If we were intelligently designed then, yes, there is room for improvement, but if we were still intimately in touch with and evolving in our native environment then we would not need to depend so heavily on sunscreen, corrective lenses, and orthopedic surgeons. If we lived in our natural environment our skin would be used to the sun, the full use of our eyes would not lead to nearsightedness, and the natural movements of joints would make joint replacements a rare necessity.

What I want to reiterate here is that evolution in the natural world creates strong species that are well adapted to that world. In a way, humans are so smart that they found a way around the relentlessness of evolution. Our intellect has allowed us to become the most dominant species on Earth. However, it is also weakening the strong genes that millions of years of evolution created. Further, it has slowed the already super-slow evolutionary process. Slowing the evolutionary process, while at the same time continuing to increase the rate of change in our environment and way of life, is a recipe for disaster. Our failing health is just the first warning sign of what is to come.

I will end this chapter with a prescient analysis by Rene Dubos. In the research article, *"Natural Environments, Ancestral Diets, and Microbial Ecology: Is There a Modern 'Paleo-Deficit Disorder? Part 1,"* A.C. Logan and co-authors discuss the work of Dubos in regards to what he saw going on around him and warnings he had for the future:

> Dubos argued that because humans are very adaptable, the relationship between an evolutionary mismatch and erosion of health would be stealth-like; there would be only minimal awareness of the association, especially early on in the era of technology and urbanization. [...] Moreover, since humans are also attracted to gadgets and, as Dubos argued, "seem to accept willingly, and indeed enjoy" many of the biological stresses of mega city life, it would be even more difficult to appreciate

ancestral needs that might be missed in the modern environment. [....] The detrimental health effects of the slow and insidious presence of physical and psychological toxins, disturbed circadian rhythms, artificial foodstuffs (all acting in concert with the absence of nature interaction), would bypass identification by most individuals—rather, according to Dubos, they would only be apparent in the overall health statistics of the larger nature-disconnected population over time.

During his lifetime, Dubos brought much attention to what harm we humans are bringing on ourselves. He died in 1982. Yet, it doesn't seem that we listened, and we have done exactly what Dubos suggested we would. What is it going to take for us to realize what we are doing? What happens to a species that does not pick up on the early signs of its demise? What happens to a species that stops adapting to the environment it is living in?

Chapter 11: A Twenty-First Century Oregon Trail

Despite how much I enjoyed Portland I decided it was time to leave once school was over. I had great friends out there; it was a great city that at times felt like a small town, and I even had a job lined up after graduation, but I just couldn't shake the feeling that I should move on. If there was one thing that told me that staying in Oregon was not meant to be, it was a trip back there after vacationing with my family on the coast of North Carolina. The plan was to get back and start my new job within the next month, but this trip changed my mind.

I was flying from Wilmington, NC to Portland and had layovers in Charlotte and Phoenix. When I got to the terminal in Wilmington I learned that there were two flights going to Charlotte. The one that wasn't mine was cancelled and there was a huge line of people at the desk trying to get on my flight. I sat on the plane for an hour while they tried to get as many people on as they could. If we stayed much longer I would be in danger of missing my next flight. We finally took off and were on our way to Charlotte.

After we landed we were halfway to the gate when the pilot stopped the plane and said over the intercom that there was lightening in the area and that all planes had been grounded. Since there was a plane at our gate we had to stay parked somewhere between the runway and the gate. The captain assured us that we would all make our connecting flights because all the other planes weren't going anywhere either. We sat on the plane for almost two hours while the lightening passed over us.

When we finally got into the airport, I ran to my next flight and just made it. I was surprised that they were taking off so quickly, considering so many people were delayed and trying to get to their flights. I was finally off to Phoenix and was starting to question if I even wanted to go back to the West Coast at all.

I had already missed my connecting flight in Phoenix because of the lightening fiasco in Charlotte but was hoping that there was another flight that night that I could get on. There wasn't. The next flight was at 7:00 AM the next morning. It was currently around 7:30 PM, and since these delays were not the fault of the airline, no hotel was offered. Being a poor student I decided to stay in the airport overnight.

Apparently Sunday night is vacuuming night at the Phoenix airport and they don't miss a spot. It must also be policy not to skip an area of the floor just because someone is sleeping on it. It felt like those vacuums got dangerously close to my face while I laid there with my eye closed. I'm surprised they didn't kick me and ask me to move.

Seven AM finally rolled around. I was hoping to get a little vacuum-free sleep on the plane to Portland. Everything seemed like it was finally on track until about 20 minutes into the flight when the captain came on and said that there was a mechanical problem with the plane. It wasn't a big deal but since this airline had no mechanics in Portland they would have to turn around and head back to Phoenix. The whole trip was beginning to seem like a modern day, absurd Oregon Trail—if your plane didn't get cancelled, and the lightening and the vacuum cleaners didn't prematurely end your journey, then maybe the mechanical malfunctions would. At least I wasn't on the original Oregon Trail because with the kind of luck I was having I would have broken many axles, lost the wagon fording a river, and probably died of dysentery. At this point I really wondered if I should go back to Oregon, as it all felt like a clear sign that I was not meant to go.

We got back to Phoenix and sat on the plane for an hour while they tried to fix it only for them to finally decide that we needed a new plane. We all unloaded and then loaded onto a new plane at a different gate. By the time I finally made it back to Portland I decided it was time to leave. Three days later I got offered a job in Ireland and took it without hesitation.

On that trip back to Oregon it felt like I probably could have driven back quicker than it took me to fly. About a month later I did exactly that, only in the opposite direction. I had some things that I wanted to store at my parents' house while I went to work in Ireland and decided to rent a small moving truck and drive across the country. My dad flew out to Portland to drive back with me and we decided to stop along the way and make a trip out of it by seeing some sights.

We went to Crater Lake, drove through Las Vegas, and saw the Grand Canyon before running into some trouble at Hoover Dam. Okay, so it wasn't really trouble, but there was a moment or two where I was worried. As we were driving up to the dam we saw a few signs that said "NO COMMERCIAL VEHICLES." I didn't really think about it because while we were in a moving truck, it wasn't "commercial." As we waited in the line of cars I watched people get checked and then make their way through. When it was almost our turn we were instructed to pull over to the side.

A man in a military outfit approached the window, and I rolled it down. He said trucks like this are not allowed on the dam. I briefly told him that I was just moving across the country and that we wanted to stop and see the dam. All he said was, "Could you please step out of the vehicle?" My heartbeat increased a little as I got out. He asked me to open the back so he could see what we were transporting. I immediately started going through the inventory thinking of things that could be interpreted as threatening. Turns out a beat-up bike, some golf clubs, and a model spine from chiropractic school were things the military didn't find threatening either.

I closed up the truck and he told me I could return to my vehicle. For a second I thought he was going to let us through but then he told us to loop around and go back out the way we came. My dad and I were left wondering why he asked to see what was in the truck if he was just going to turn us around anyway. Guess it just wasn't meant to be.

We salvaged what we could by heading up to the lookout over Lake Mead. It was much more beautiful than I anticipated. I had never seen a lake that color of blue. I wondered if it was because I was used to seeing lakes surrounded by green while this one was surrounded by the brown of the desert, and it really brought out the lakes eyes, if you know what I mean. We also stopped at an overlook that opened onto the Colorado River a little further down from the dam. It wasn't too impressive—just some brown mountains. I had never been to the desert before and it amazed me how dead it looked. I knew there was life on it but couldn't help but wonder if the dam had affected life downstream and kept thinking that this view I was looking at wasn't "meant to be" like this.

My dad took over driving and I decided to do some research on my phone about the affects the dam has had on the land and wildlife. Turns out that wildlife above the dam flourished but the same could not be said for below the dam. Since being built it has eroded a lot of land, resulted in declines in populations of species, like the endangered desert tortoise, and has caused populations of trout and salmon to decrease substantially.

The Hoover Dam is one impressive display of how humans have become masters of altering the natural environment to make life easier for them. However, scientists and engineers now realize the impacts it has had. The dam is just one way in which we have used our smarts to decrease the hardships of life. While I care about how our natural world is affected by things like the Hoover Dam, I would like to draw attention to the parallel of us continuing to change our way of life the way we have. If we continue on this path it will lead to consequences that affect humans the same way the Hoover Dam has affected the land and wildlife below it on the Colorado River.

Chapter 12: Our Plot of Heather: The Choice is Ours

"Though nature grants vast periods of time for the work of natural selection, she does not grant an indefinite period; for as all organic beings are striving, it may be said, to seize on each place in the economy of nature, if any one species does not become modified and improved in a corresponding degree with its competitors, it will soon be exterminated."

—Charles Darwin

Once we realize that we are indeed slowing our evolutionary process, the words of Darwin quoted above, written in 1859, become quite haunting. By now you are probably seeing that I think humans, and most species on the planet, are doomed because of the world that humans have created. While I do think we face big issues, I remain cautiously optimistic about the future of our species. We will get into why in Part Three.

Notice that I didn't say the earth is in danger, just the many species that inhabit it. Earth has survived many dramatic changes in environment and the rise and fall of many life forms, so I'm not too worried about the earth. To a certain extent, the only reason that humans care about climate change, shrinking ecosystems, polluted oceans, and the loss of so many species in recent history is because these changes are creating a world that is not compatible with the life that has evolved on it, including us.

We are realizing that, as a species, we are changing our environment too fast. Species that are dying are essential to keeping the earth operating the way it is right now, which is the only way of operation we are completely sure we ourselves can survive. We are also slowly getting the idea that over the last 10,000 years we have lost a lot of our genetic resiliency through the attack of the modern world on our genes and through the passing on of those epigenetically weaker genes discussed in the previous chapter. An inhospitable environment combined with weaker genes does not bode well for us. We are evolutionarily fragile, just like every other living species, and our current way of life is amplifying that fragility.

The changes we see on our planet are in large part due to changes in the human way of life, though I also acknowledge that the earth went through many periods of heating and cooling, along with many massive environmental changes, before humans even got here. So, while I believe we are accelerating a climate situation that we would be wise to try to mitigate, we could never stop environmental change as a whole; it's inevitable over time on Earth. Many people are so passionate and determined to slow the change of the planet. Yet even if we cease the human causes, we won't escape climate change forever—possibly not even for a very long time. Because of this, and because we know deep down that we have lost the genetic resiliency to deal with such inevitable changes, the better approach to creating a healthier world and healthier humans is to focus on lifestyle changes that will create the strongest genes in ourselves that we can.

So humans are heading down a scary road, but aside from failing health, what else can we expect if we stay on this path? The answer is not fun to talk about. In his book, *Collapse,* Jared Diamond discusses many past societies that did themselves in. When discussing the fall of the people of Easter Island he says, "The collapse of Easter society followed swiftly upon the society's reaching its peak of population, monument construction, and environmental impact." He would come to similar conclusions when looking at the collapse of the Anasazi and Maya societies as well.

Based on Diamond's observations, if we want to learn from past societies, we should be careful not to meet or exceed the planet's population limit...oops. We should also be careful not to build too much at the expense of our limited resources...oops. Lastly, we should not live in such a way that it has a detrimental effect on the environment we call home. Oops! To be fair, we didn't have the warning of scientists like Diamond until very recently. Now that we can look at the world through an evolutionary lens, we can try to predict what will happen if we continue living the way we are. The difference between us and those past societies is that we have gained enough knowledge to do something about it. Our intellect may be enough to bail us out, but only if we play our cards right.

It is important to note that Easter Island was especially vulnerable because it is the most remote island in the world. When the islanders exhausted their resources and put themselves in dire straits, they had nowhere to go, and they didn't have the technology to leave. We are fast approaching a situation similar to what happened on Easter Island, only on a global scale. There are hardly any pristine islands to which we can escape the conditions we have created. Western waste is literally rolling in with the tide onto the shores of San Blas. Within this context, the quote referenced in Chapter 6 by Elizabeth Kolbert bears repeating: "A species that needs to migrate to keep up with rising temperatures, but is trapped in a forest fragment—even a very large forest fragment—is a species that isn't likely to make it." We, effectively, are trapping ourselves in a planet-sized forest fragment. I only hope that we can use our smarts and broader knowledge to navigate out of our situation before the earth becomes an uninhabitable trap just as Easter Island became for its inhabitants.

In addition to not being able to adapt to our changing environment, there is another consequence of weakened genes that puts our species in danger. In the last fifty years fertility rates have halved among humans globally.[1] It has even become a specialty of rising popularity among doctors as infertility clinics are growing in numbers. This decrease in fertility can be attributed to our change in environment. In his exhaustive study of the natural world, Darwin noticed the same outcomes in other species:

> I have more than once alluded to a large body of facts, which I have collected, showing that when animals and plants are removed from their natural conditions, they are extremely liable to have their reproductive systems seriously affected. This, in fact, is the great bar to the domestication of animals.

Not only does this suggest that removing ourselves from the natural world in which we evolved may be a reason why infertility is on the rise, but it also forces us to accept that we are a domesticated version of our wild ancestors—just as dogs are domesticated versions of wolves.

Infertility is sometimes mistakenly thought to be only a female problem, but sperm count and viability have dropped off significantly in the recent past.[2] Darwin once made the observation that when it comes to reproduction in species taken from their natural environment, "the male element is the most liable to be affected."

I believe that this increase in infertility is a direct result of the combination of our rapidly changing environment and our weakening genes. The lifestyle changes that make the body too weak to create a pregnancy are the same ones that led to the unnatural human environment we talked about in Chapter 8. Darwin says it best yet again:

> When organic beings are placed during several generations under conditions not natural to them, they are extremely liable to vary, which is due, as I believe, to their reproductive systems having been specifically affected, though in a lesser degree than when sterility ensues.

I believe Darwin's words describe exactly the state of human fertility today—it has been largely affected, but we are not yet sterile. Infertility is just another symptom of being too far removed from the natural environment of humans. If we stay on this path, we can only expect infertility numbers to grow until they result in huge drops in population due to the inability to procreate. While tragic, this may not be entirely a bad thing, given the dire situation we are in. Humans are struggling in the world we have created to such an extent that growing numbers of people are not strong enough to create or support a pregnancy, which, in the natural world, is the primary purpose of life.

I saw an excellent video at the American Museum of Natural History in New York City which demonstrates how it took humans around 200,000 years to get to 1 billion people but it has only taken us 200 years to go from 1 billion to 7 billion. (At the time of this writing, you can see this video by searching "human population through time" on the American Museum of Natural History YouTube channel). It makes sense that modern agriculture and advancements in medical science have been the main reason for this massive growth in the last 200 years, because in nature, food scarcity and health are limiting factors when it comes to population growth. If you remove those, you get exponential growth.

We may be the only species in the history of life as we know it that has become so successful at surviving and also has the intelligence needed to consider that we may need to change our definition of success. In most all species, sexual behavior has evolved to ensure that we procreate and pass on genes. That strong desire for us to have sex is there for a reason; how successful could we be at surviving and passing on genes otherwise? This deeply ingrained desire would be difficult to halt just by convincing ourselves that the world is overpopulated. Yet, if we don't find a solution, we may find ourselves asking difficult questions about restricting the number of children we have and what happens then when "illegal" children are born.

Another problem with this exponential growth is that, once people are born, the socioeconomic system we have set up may fail to meet their basic needs. This is evident in nature because when a species is in ideal conditions it multiplies to the greatest numbers it can, such as rats becoming more abundant in a trash-filled city and crops producing more yields when fertilizer is used. On the flip side, there are many limiting factors in nature that keep a species from growing to excessive numbers. It has been observed that mice in the wild lose pregnancies when there is not enough food. Since humans have removed themselves from these limiting factors of nature, we have many people on the planet living lives of starvation and poverty.

It might seem like a humanitarian approach to attempt to give each and every person the same opportunities that the most privileged people have. I don't think that is such a good idea—our world is suffering the repercussions of us living the way we do, and those of us living a Western lifestyle put the most strain on our struggling world. If we tried to give everyone on earth the same things that we in the United States enjoy then I believe two things would happen: first, we would just continue to create more and more people and, just like now, we would not be able to provide the growing numbers with the same standards of living, which would in turn create more people living in poverty and starvation. Secondly, our Earth would become uninhabitable for us, due to the complete exhaustion of its resources and widespread pollution, leading, ultimately, to the extinction of our species. So you see, the Western approach is not humanitarian, and it likely will lead to pain and suffering in greater numbers of people and could very well lead to the end of humans.

Back in Chapter 6 we discussed some important principles of evolution. Applying them to humans can help us understand where we are heading. However, applying evolution to humans in this sense is uncomfortable and we must tread with care. In the natural process of evolution, the less fit beings do not survive to pass on their genes. Over time this allows for the strengthening of the genes of the species as only the fittest genes are passed on. Before you get mad and think that I am saying we should allow the poor and starving to die, which I would never suggest, let's take a deeper look at this process.

Humans have created a world where the "fittest" members of our species are not those with the genes best fit for the environment. In our capitalistic society the fittest are the members of the species with the highest socioeconomic status. A recent study that looked at life expectancy found that there was a gap of more than 20 years between the most affluent and most impoverished counties in the United States.[3] Competition involved in today's evolutionary process is largely affected by socioeconomic status rather than how fit genes may be for the environment. This is just another way humans have begun to defy the laws of nature.

Someone born socioeconomically advantaged today could have the most unfit genes ever, yet because they are affluent, they don't have to worry too much about getting to pass on their genes. The fact that they could not make it very far in the natural world is of no consequence. Conversely, someone born in the poorest country in the world may have the fittest genes we have ever seen, yet they may not get the opportunity to pass them on because of the hardships they may face. Socioeconomic inequality is negatively affecting our evolution.

We are faced with some harsh realities. Trying to give everyone the luxuries of the West would exacerbate our problems, but if we let evolution take its course we will continue to see the death of human beings just because of where they are born. How is anyone supposed to decide what to do? I don't want to see human beings suffer, but I also don't what to see the destruction of our species. Rene Dubos said that, "To save people from death by measures of public health is proving to be relatively easy, but no solution is in sight for the many problems created by their survival." We can only hope that a solution will present itself in time. I will do my best to share one approach with you by the end of this book, but first, let's learn a way nature self-regulates when confronted with the issue of population control.

In *The Selfish Gene,* Dawkins tells us about the red grouse, a bird that eats the heather plant. Early in the season the males fight over large plots of heather, often securing more than they could ever eat. The losers seem to "accept" that they are not going to secure a plot of food and become outcasts, who by the end of the season, starve to death. The losers are still perfectly capable of breeding, proven by the fact that if one of the plot owners is killed during the season then one of the losers takes over his plot and breeds, but they do not breed unless this happens. It is almost as if these birds know that the result of overcrowding would not be in the best interest of the species as a whole—almost like the losers do not breed because they know their offspring would suffer. If they bred they would be likely to lose many offspring, and it is better for them to wait and hope that a plot of heather becomes available, so that is what they do. The human species may not be able to mimic this kind of self-sacrifice on a grand scale, but if we can recalibrate the way we look at our own plots of heather, I believe there is a way forward.

I especially believe this because there is evidence that humans in the recent past were much more conscious about reproduction. Dr. Weston Price spent much of his life studying the dietary and lifestyle habits of traditional people. He talks at length about how traditional people practiced child spacing and honored specific diets or foods for those couples attempting to conceive. They did this to limit overpopulation within a group and ensure health of the children. Sally Fallon Morell, who has spent her life spreading the message of Dr. Prices' work, discusses modern day reproductive practices critically saying:

> We are very careless in the way we bring children into the world, and when something goes wrong, we blame it on one of the three G's—germs, genes, or God. Traditional cultures knew better; they knew that the responsibility for bringing healthy children into the world rested squarely on their shoulders.

Recent science has even confirmed that the traditional people were wise to practice more conscious child bearing. Research has shown that there are definite health benefits to spacing out children and that the ideal interval between childbirths is at least 18 months.[4]

We must continue to search for ways to alter the troublesome future of humans suggested by our declining health and overpopulation. Obviously, we as humans cannot decide which humans are less "fit" and do away with them—this is horrifying. Anyway, only nature has the mechanism to determine which individuals are fit. Also, because there are way too many of us now, we all can't just go back to how humans used to live before the Agricultural Revolution without destroying our natural world even more. We have created quite the predicament for ourselves, and finding a way out of it will take some ingenuity and hard work—not just by activists, researchers, and governments, but by each and every one of us.

While I don't know that the situations in this chapter will progress to their dystopic conclusions in my lifetime, thinking about them is still scary. I hope that humanity comes together to forge a better path so that we don't get to a point where we must address these possible futures head on in the present. Unfortunately, it seems that this is where we are headed. Because of the dramatic changes and rapid advancement of humans in the last 10,000 years, we must confront these uncomfortable questions. In order to work toward solutions, we must become comfortable talking about them and taking into account the evolutionary way of the natural world. Fortunately, I believe that we can each individually look within ourselves to do something about it while simultaneously achieving better health, which is the subject of Part Three. The solutions I present do not provide every answer, but they are fairly simple steps that each one of us can take. If we take them, we will not only be storing up our own individual plots of heather—we will also be contributing to the restoration of a more natural, ecologically-aware way of life.

Part Three: The Selfish Solution

Chapter 13: Girl on a Train

After three months in Ireland, I had finally gotten over the shock of being a resident in another country instead of just a visitor. I had settled into my routine and was on the 20-minute Luas (Dublin commuter rail) to work, a little outside of the city of Dublin. I was still building up a patient base and didn't have a full schedule yet, so I grew accustomed to sharing the journey with only a few others, as I rarely went during busy morning commute hours.

About halfway through my ride, a man pushing a woman in a wheelchair joined me and an elderly man on the nearly empty train. Their toddler was sticking close behind them. I could tell they weren't regular riders because after a few minutes they started wondering if they were on the right train. They were, in fact, on the wrong train, headed to Saggart instead of to Tallaght. They consulted the old man, who told them that they should get off at the next stop—where he was also getting off—and take the very next train to come along.

At the next stop, they all exited, the couple making sure that they had their toddler in tow. Right as they got off the train the toddler turned around and spotted something left behind—her stuffed animal. She ran to it just as the doors of the train started to close. With her prized possession in her grasp, she turned to see the man and woman (her parents, I assumed) moving away from her on the platform outside. I didn't notice there was an emergency stop button until weeks later.

My guess is that the driver was not looking at his cameras, because the train continued to move right on schedule. I approached the girl who was now scared and crying. I asked for her name but I couldn't understand what she said through her sobbing. She was endearing, trying to tell me the whole story, unaware that I saw the whole thing. I remember thinking how trusting she was of me, a total stranger.

I had to think quickly. I knew her parents' plans were to get on the next train, but that was before they were separated from their daughter. I decided to convince her to get off at the next stop with me. She did not take to this idea as well as she had taken to talking to me. She backed away from the doors as we slowed for the next stop. I kept telling her that I wanted to help her, and we needed to get off here. The doors opened, and I stood halfway out of the door asking her to come with me. The doors tried to close, and I stopped them. I guess the doors trying to close made her think that she might end up on the train all alone, or maybe she figured that her parents went out that way so maybe she would find them out there. Either way, she decided to come with me.

Once on the platform, another train came by, headed the other way, and the girl got really scared and grabbed my leg. I took this as an opportunity to scoop her up to be sure she didn't run off. At this point I really didn't know what to do. Should I take her back to the last stop? Should I wait and hope that they showed up on the next train? I decided to wait for the next train, and if that didn't work, I would take her back to the last stop. It seemed like an hour until the next train came through, though it was probably 5-10 minutes. The girl went through a cycle of louder and softer crying, and I just hoped she wouldn't change her mind about me and start trying to run away.

To my relief I saw the next train arriving. I would have given anything at that point for her parents to be on it. In the meantime I thought of a new plan: if they were not on the train I would run up to tell the driver of the situation. When the train pulled up to the platform, there were her parents, her mother in tears and her father with determination and worry all over his face. When they saw us their expression immediately changed, and I am guessing the girl saw them too, because she almost jumped out of my arms.

I hurried on to the train, which was a little more crowded than the last one. This meant that this reunion would have an audience. They were, of course, so relieved and so thankful. They told me that when the next train had pulled up they went to the driver and told him what had happened. Apparently, he radioed to the driver ahead of him, updated him, and asked him to check his train at the next stop for a young girl. The driver said that he had seen the girl follow me off the train at his last stop; my guess is that my blocking the doors had caused him to look at his cameras to see what was going on. I told her parents, Rachael and Eamonn, that they must have been terrified to know that she got off at the next stop with a complete stranger. At this point they didn't seem to care; they had her back and that was all that mattered. I rode with them until my stop, where we said our goodbyes, and I was off to work.

About a year later I picked up a book by Richard Dawkins, called *The Selfish Gene*. He talks a lot about altruism in this book and about why it does not necessarily come naturally in humans. The selfish pursuit to further one's own genes and no one else's has been the impulse of life for a very long time. This made me wonder about my experience on the train. While I think that we are primarily programmed to be selfish, the countless selfless acts done by humans every day prove that we have evolved a sense of altruism as well. Evolutionarily speaking, I think we are in a time when we go back and forth between our selfish and altruistic ways.

We haven't really gotten to a point where we can depend on our altruism to solve the world's problems. The selfish drive is still strong and arguably winning. Because of this, I think the only choice for our survival is to learn how we can leverage our selfish impulses to achieve health and save our species.

Chapter 14: Playing to Our Strengths

"Let us try to teach generosity and altruism, because we are born selfish. Let us understand what our own selfish genes are up to, because we may then at least have the chance to upset their designs, something that no other species has ever aspired to do."

—Richard Dawkins

Humans are the only species that we know of to become powerful enough to change the earth at such a global extent. Encouragingly, we are also the only species smart enough to realize that our trajectory may not be in our best interest or in the best interest of the ecosystem we depend on. The problem is that not enough of us are doing something about it. This is not surprising considering we are selfishly wired by evolution to put our individual needs and the needs of our offspring first. Being the dominant species on an earth that supports the life of predominantly selfish species makes us the most successfully selfish species on the planet. Congratulations! Although it is generally seen as a negative trait in our society, I think it is time to liberate selfishness from its negative connotations, because I believe that we can use it to our advantage to erase our health epidemic and protect the planet.

First, we will consider the perspective of Richard Dawkins in his book, *The Selfish Gene,* to make some sense of our selfish nature. Dawkins illustrated that our genes are really pulling the strings. After all, genes are what survive through the generations, whereas individuals do not. He makes the compelling argument that all living things are just vessels to harbor genes until they can be passed on to the next generation of vessels. I am picturing the scene at the end of *Men in Black* when you find out that a little alien had been in the skull of that human, piloting it all along. While that is just an analogy, it is an interesting thought experiment to think of living individuals as the middlemen our genes use to gain information about the environment so that they can be in fitter individuals in the next generation.

Natural selection sculpts our genes across generations, allowing us to survive despite shifting environmental conditions. Dawkins says our genes create individuals based on "conditions of past gene survival." In other words, each individual's genetic instructions were written over many, many generations before. Dawkins provides the example of polar bears. These bears have lived in cold, snowy climates for a long time, and their genes know that and give them thick white fur that will keep them warm and camouflaged, enhancing the likelihood they will survive to pass on genes. But imagine if the environment changes quickly and the polar bear finds itself in a warm and green place. Suddenly its genetic inheritance would put the bear at a huge disadvantage, because polar bear genes would still be creating polar bears with thick white fur. This would be like making a substantial business decision based on your numbers from a decade ago instead of the previous year. Evolution enables species to survive, but only via slow change over many generations. As you know by now, this book presents the argument that this example with the polar bear is already happening with many species on the planet, including humans.

A similar example is with humans and sweets. We have evolved a taste—almost an addiction—for sweet things. This might have been advantageous to us back when sweet foods were not very plentiful, because when we did come across them, gorging on them would have given us a sharp increase in energy and stores of excess energy in fat cells for the winter. But since we did not come across these foods often, we have mainly evolved to eat fat as an energy source. For most of the year we were much better off eating a high fat diet. This is why today we find that carbohydrates make us gain weight and fat does not. As we have increased our sugar and grain intake and removed ourselves from our environment's impact on our ability to survive, we have also seen a breakdown in health. Our genes are programming us the best they know how, but we have made their job impossible by rapidly and continuously changing our way of life.

Just like a desire for sweet foods developed in us, one of the most dominate characteristics that genes have developed through uncountable generations of life are selfish characteristics. In his book, Dawkins discusses the ins and outs of many of these characteristics seen in species throughout the natural world. Humans are no exception and, through trying to predict what will give a living thing advantages to survive, our genes have programmed us to selfishly put the survival of ourselves and our children—and therefore the individual genes we harbor—above everything else.

For millions of years the human gene's best chance of being passed on was to instruct us to look out for ourselves and do whatever necessary to ensure the survival of our genetic line. It was only in the last 10,000 years that we started practicing how to get along while living in large numbers. We still need practice at this relatively new characteristic. In general, large groups of humans are pretty slow to come together, agree on an action, and then pursue it, because we haven't been doing that sort of thing for very long. For the most part, the selfishness of securing our own genes' survival comes first and cooperation with others for the survival of the species comes second because that has been evolutionarily ingrained in us.

I would guess that this is part of the reason that the majority of people do not show interest in acting in unselfish ways. As negative as this sounds, if you ask most people to take a day off work to participate in a march for a humanitarian cause or to volunteer in another city recovering from disaster, most would say no because they have to work to provide for their family. Don't be mad at them—they are just doing what life on this planet has been doing since it began. On the flip side, we celebrate those who commit unselfish acts because we realize the strength it can take to put aside the selfish impulses that are embedded in all of us.

In Chapter 12 I proposed that in today's world, evolutionary "fitness" doesn't have much to do with genes making us fit for our environment anymore, but rather, with the socioeconomic status that we are born into. Some argue that money is the culprit here, because if we didn't have money then we would have a more equal world. I would argue that inequality arises because the selfish drive we see in the natural world is exacerbated by the existence of money, which allows power and advantage to be horded, not only in a present moment, but also across time. In nature, we see that selfish drive in competition among animals that live in groups. Typically, an alpha male will get his pick of food and—through means including female preference and male coercion—reproductive partners. If you introduce money into this system, suddenly those who are advantaged at one point in time can exploit the situation for their future selves and children. That exploitation is perhaps even intrinsic (and therefore unavoidable) in such a system. Life has been competing for the upper hand for all of its time on Earth. Humans are no different in that we are hardwired to be selfish, too. Truly, we made it to where we are now because we are selfish. It's really hard to override billions of years of evolution.

Asking a person that has been genetically programmed over millions of years to be selfish to take personal time, money, and resources away from themselves and their families in order to "save the planet" is like asking Fido to be nicer to the mailman for the sake of the postal system. Not going to happen. If we were to take a pessimistic look at this, we may see it as a major barrier to saving ourselves and creating a healthier planet. However, just as we have used the selfish characteristics that our genes have given us to create the problems that face our species in the world today, I believe that we can use those same characteristics to solve them. If we can turn our weakness into strength and play to that strength, I think we have a chance. Mastery of our selfish nature could get us out of the mess that success put us in. Let me explain.

My passion is health, and I have spent many years of my life on a search to find what creates health in humans. However, I never expected to discover that the answer to restoring health in individual humans could also be the salvation of our species. If masses of people on Earth made changes in their own lifestyles, it would have a direct positive impact on their individual health and the health of their children, and we would see a reversal of many of the problems we are facing as a planet.

This means that, as individuals, we can stop thinking of how to tackle the overwhelming problem of the global environment and instead just look at the problems we have in each of our individual environments. As a species, if we try to tackle every issue we see in this world, it starts to seem impossible. Doing so can even contribute to poor health in the individual. It can become frustrating trying to recruit others to help fix those problems, as they either get annoyed with us or overwhelmed along with us, especially when piled on to the busy lives people already lead. If we frame the salvation of our planet and our species in a way that will allow people to make their lives better, then we *save* two birds with one stone. So in a way I am asking people to be selfish. I want people to focus on making changes in their lives that will result in better health for themselves. This task doesn't seem as daunting, so more people would be likely to make changes. In addition, just like we discussed in Chapter 4, it removes the focus from the ambiguous "them" who are destroying our lives and places it squarely on ourselves.

When it comes to campaigns like "save the whales," we can't see that the whales are dying as a result of the unfit world we have made for them. Plus, does it make sense to try and save them while completely ignoring the fact that we are struggling with our health in that same unfit environment? Changing our individual environment impacts the global environment. We can focus on ourselves and simultaneously "save the whales."

For example, if I were to ask most people if they would like to donate money to combat environmental pollution or sacrifice their weekend to protest GMOs, then I am not likely to get a lot of yeses. However, if I were to encourage people to switch to all organic food, it would have manifold positive effects. It would not only increase the amount of nutrients they get and dramatically decrease the amount of toxins they are exposed to—two things that help protect against disease—it would also decrease their exposure to the giant human experimental trial of genetically modified food. People are more likely to say yes to this suggestion to improve their health, but may not recognize that choosing organic food also combats the unsustainable practices we have developed in our agricultural system and bucks against GMOs, helping us to slow the modification of genetic information in our food.

If everyone switched to organic foods, we would feel so much better[1]; pesticides would no longer be pumped into the environment, and the cost of organic food would go down because more suppliers would be forced to adapt to our demands. Similarly, if consumers refused to bring products that use heavy metals into their personal environments, then companies would be forced to take heavy metals out of their products, which in turn would create drastic improvements in the health of individuals and the environment.

I'm sure we could imagine almost endless examples of this. In the next chapter I will detail the best ways we can change our lives to attain greater health, and I will also touch on how each change has an impact on a global scale. This is my vision of how to use my passion to better the world we live in. We have so much power. If we start to use our selfish tendencies to, in a way, overpower them, then I think the world would be radically different from what we see today.

Chapter 15: Salina Turda

While in Ireland, I took numerous trips to Romania to see my Hungarian girlfriend, Kinga, who is now my wife. Confused yet? I often daydreamed of seeing dragons, because Ron's older brother worked with dragons in Romania in the Harry Potter books. Not the best information to base my hopes on, I know, but I could still hope!

On one trip, Kinga and I travelled about 45 minutes outside of Cluj Napoca (where she was in school) to a salt mine in the Transylvanian mountains that was open for tours. She and her friends seemed to think it would be a good idea for us to go, though I wasn't exactly sure why. I was often stuck interpreting the tone of their Hungarian conversations, though Kinga did explain the important things to me in English.

The entrance to Salina Turda is a huge tunnel going into the side of a large mountain. Just outside is a ticket booth, much like I used to see outside of the county fair in my hometown. When we arrived, we paid for our tickets and headed into the dark tunnel. If I had known this place was ranked by *Business Insider* as one of the top ten "coolest underground places in the world" I might have been a little more excited, but at the time I was just following the crowd, expecting to see some old abandoned salt mines and learn a little about salt mining.

The access tunnel seemed to go on forever. It was slightly sloped, taking us deeper into the mountain. At one point the walls changed from rock to a crystal-like material. It was strange staring into the wall, because it was sort of see-through, but thick and never ending, so you could only see about a foot into the wall. It felt like something could emerge from it without being seen until the last second. It was kind of creepy. My guess was that this material was salt but I never got an answer that wasn't mostly in another language, so I'm still not sure.

The first chamber we came to was about the size of a 3-bedroom house but twice as high. There was a "crivac," a large wooden device dating back to 1881, which was used to lift big salt rocks. This room was impressive and a little bigger than anything I expected to see, but boy, was I in for more.

We made our way through other tunnels and down stairwells until we came to a small open area. On the far, upper wall there was a space of about 3-4 feet where people were looking out over the edge at something. They reminded me of scientists peering into an experimental chamber. When we got to the same spot, I was surprised to find that it opened out onto a huge cylindrical room that went way down deeper into the mine. At the bottom there was a small lake with an island in the middle that looked like three circles of land that had been joined together. I also saw boats with people in them slowly gliding on the lake. It was incredible. This room was called the Terezia mine and was 295' high and 285' in diameter. People were walking around on the island, and I was eager to get down there—but there was more.

We went down many switch-back steps made of wood that let us out onto a boardwalk. As we rounded the corner I realized that the boardwalk went around the entire perimeter of another extremely large rectangular-shaped room, its bottom a long way below us. This was the Rudolf mine, and it is 137' deep, 154' wide, and 262' long. This room had a basketball court, ping-pong tables, an amphitheater, a playground, and, most impressive of all, a giant Ferris wheel right in the center. The whole room was lit up by long fluorescent lights that were hanging on cables from the ceiling. I had never seen anything like it.

We crossed the boardwalk and descended 13 floors worth of steps on the opposite side of the room. It was a whole different view at the bottom. Looking up, we could see formerly hidden slanted parts of the ceiling that had thousands of salty stalactites. It was hard to hear down there because there were so many people and all the voices were bouncing off the walls and echoing everywhere.

We decided to play ping-pong. I had played with Kinga before and knew I was no match for her. Keeping score felt more like slowly counting to 21. After we finished we walked past the Ferris wheel, past a large elevator shuttling people up and down, and through a big opening with a bridge in it. The bridge led to the other large cylindrical room we had seen earlier and went over the lake to the island of conjoined circles, where we took in the sights and took a rowboat for a spin.

We eventually made our way back up and out of the mine. As we strolled to the entrance I wondered if any life could live down there. The few placards of information down in the mine were in Romanian. Once we got back to Kinga's apartment I did some research. The mine did have life! Various species of archaea and bacteria are halophilic in nature, meaning that that have adapted to conditions of extreme salinity. What fascinating creatures.

I later remembered these creatures when thinking about how humans are maladapted to the current environment society has us in. Just like a polar bear would not thrive and eventually die if it was suddenly placed in the Caribbean, and a tropical fish would struggle and die if released in a mountain stream, these little bacteria would not do so well outside of the salt mine where they lived. I wondered if there had been any creatures still alive in the salt spots on my pants by the time I got back to the apartment. When it comes to health, environment is everything.

Chapter 16: Resource Your Health

"The earth is literally our mother, not only because we depend on her for nurture and shelter but even more because the human species has been shaped by her in the womb of evolution. Our salvation depends on our ability to create a religion of nature."

– Rene Dubos

The line of thinking described in the previous chapters lead me to the realization that the answer to our health issues does not lie in new and improved treatments, the latest research, or cutting edge technology, but in the return to a more ancient lifestyle. As we discussed in Chapter 2, medical treatments cause more deaths than our leading diseases do, research is often funded by companies with an agenda, and many technologies contribute to the environmental change we are struggling to keep up with.

Don't get me wrong; I think that some treatments, research, and technology out there are fascinating and have their place when it comes to restoring the body to its optimal state. However, Max Planck tells us that, "Science cannot solve the ultimate mystery of nature. And that is because, in the last analysis, we ourselves are part of the mystery that we are trying to solve." Medical research and technology will never provide us with what we need to save ourselves unless we acknowledge that we are a part of nature, and we start conducting that science with the evolutionary laws of the natural world in mind.

I am not opposed to science and technology. However, whenever a new technology comes along we need to consider how/if it can push us further away from the natural environment in which we evolved. We need to ask how that technology will affect us in the long run. When we reach a verdict on those questions it should guide us as to whether or not we let that new technology infiltrate our lives. Unfortunately, we humans tend to maintain the status quo of our lives. We seem to think that eventually a scientific or technological advancement will come along to save us from our unsustainable lifestyles. However, avoiding the demise of our species may depend on each of us individually taking action.

Don't worry; I am not going to suggest that everyone resort to living a life in the wild. Our hunter-gatherer ancestors not only had a hard life, but also that life is not realistic for us, and at this point may cause more problems than it would fix. However, we can work to get our personal environments back in line with our ancestral environment in ways that fit within the confines of a modern lifestyle. Those of us with access to modern lifestyles live in the best of times because we can combine our own advantages with those of our ancestors. We can utilize what we have learned about how humans lived in the past to achieve better health in the modern world. Over the last 300 years or so, we have been using the tools of scientific inquiry to examine the past and present in search of answers. We can peer into every period in the history of our species to gain knowledge about ourselves. It's not only the best of both worlds—it's the best of all human worlds since our split from our common ancestry with apes.

Although modern medicine neglects to incorporate knowledge of our place in the natural world in its methods, we don't have to. I know this is true because I am proud to say that, aside from the collateral damage that is type 1 diabetes, all the inflammatory conditions I suffered with as a child are now gone for good. I did this by **re**sourcing where I attained health by altering my personal environment. This conveniently gave me the name of my health website, ResourceYourHealth.com. It took many years of trial and error and constant pursuit of knowledge but this has changed my life. I want to share with you the strategies I found most helpful, but before we delve into those I want to talk a little bit about how disease develops so that you can see why these strategies work.

The funny thing about chronic diseases is that they do not actually exist; they are just things that humans made up. There was no list of diseases that came down from the sky with a note that said, "These are the diseases of mankind, beware!" What are real are the symptoms that people feel when they are in an environment they are not well adapted to. Way back in the beginning of Western medicine, doctors started to see the same patterns of symptoms in people and decided to call each different set of symptoms a certain disease. Doctors are trained to categorize symptoms and the results of diagnostic tests in order to identify the "disease" the patient has. In medical school the classifying of symptoms into a disease is of utmost importance, because once you get the diagnosis you know what treatment (drug or surgery) to give. Our medical system is obsessed with the diagnosis. Without it doctors don't know what treatment to render and insurance companies won't pay. The diagnosis gets everyone paid but leaves the patient asking, "How did I get this disease?" The most common reply to this question is, "It's genetic."

As we have discussed, your genes are not entirely set in stone and more often than not they are not at fault for a disease. If you start to dig deep and really get to the bottom of why symptoms present themselves you can start to understand where all this disease is coming from. So let's look at how our modern environment contributes to the symptoms that can land us in the doctor's office.

Ideally, we are born into this world as a healthy baby in a healthy homeostasis. Even this is becoming a rarer occurrence, because most babies are born loaded up with toxic chemicals their mom may have come in contact with.[1] Further, we are born with the epigenetic effects that our parents and grandparents have created for us. Arguably though, when we are born, we are as clean a slate as we will ever be. Unfortunately, as we all well know, from birth we are slowly moving toward death. In between this time many, many things happen to us, and it is the combined effect of these things that will determine how fast or how slow we reach the end. Everything from what food we eat, to how many traumatic events we go through, to whether we live in an urban or rural setting—everything is either prolonging life or pushing us faster toward disease and death.

For example, let's look at what happens to many babies born in the Western medical system today. Right from the beginning, a third of babies in the U.S. are born via Cesarean section rather than naturally. Sometimes this is necessary, but reports show that 26% of Cesarean sections were not necessary but were done anyway[2]. Many times this happens because a scheduled surgery is more convenient than waiting for birth to naturally occur. Having a Cesarean section puts a child at a disadvantage when it comes to living a symptom-free life. In natural birth, the baby is exposed to bacterium in the birth canal, which inoculates their gut and ensures proper immune function and digestion. Further, bacteria from the biologic mother are specific to her and allow the baby to best digest her breast milk for maximal nutritional benefits. Any interruption in this process can contribute to health issues later in life.

To further compromise the development of a child's immune function and digestion, many babies are fed formula instead of breast milk. Aside from being the ultimate nutrition for the child, especially if their mom has access to a nutrient-rich diet, breast milk also contains colostrum. Colostrum is what completes the sealing off of the lining of the digestive tract so that bad things don't get in. It gives the baby the immunoglobulins needed to develop an immune system that can fight off invaders. The majority of the body's immune system is located in aspects of the digestive system, so if the baby wasn't a natural birth and wasn't breastfed, we have to assume that their immune system and digestive system is not optimally functional. To add insult to injury, every child is then given many vaccinations within the first few years of life. These vaccinations are reliant on a properly functioning immune system. I am not going to suggest that we should or should not vaccinate children. Society today seems to want to label anyone who questions vaccines as anti-vaccine. I am not anti-vaccine, but I am pro-vaccine choice and pro-vaccine safety.

From there, as they grow up and become adults, many children do not eat a nutrient-rich diet, which leads to them getting sick and taking many doses of unnecessary antibiotics. They will also come in contact with an unavoidable and uncountable amount of toxins throughout their life, and they will be over stressed from the high speed, non-stop chase for money and survival that is today's society. At any point during this time, depending on the hardiness of their genes, their bodies could be giving them signals that they are in a bad environment through symptoms like headaches, fatigue, frequent colds, and irritability, but nothing that our medical system really considers worth attention. Although the timing depends on the hardiness of their genes, one day they end up with a full-blown Western medicine ICD 10 certified diagnosis. Most people are blindsided by this diagnosis, when in reality their body was giving them warning signs all along. Now they end up in the medical system that kills more people per year than heart disease or cancer. The insanity must stop.

On a more personal note, I was not a natural birth, I was partially breast fed, and I was fully vaccinated. Those things, along with the poor diet I was eating and the anxious child that I was, lead me to the inflammatory childhood I experienced. My gut was very inflamed and my immune system was very dysfunctional, which eventually resulted in my autoimmune disease, type 1 diabetes. This was not my fault. It was not my parents fault, and it was not my doctor's fault. This was a result of me growing up in a society that is completely out of touch with its natural environment. My body was trying to let me, my parents, and my doctors know how out of touch I was with my natural environment; we just didn't know how to read the signs.

To further illustrate how disease develops, I like to use the phrase "death by a thousand cuts." Every little thing you come in contact with that has a negative effect on your health is a cut. Some things make bigger cuts than others. Everyone has a different cut limit that their body can withstand before showing symptoms, as determined by the hardiness of our genes. We could probably never rid ourselves of all of these cuts. However, if we eliminate as many of them as we can, especially the bigger ones, we will significantly increase our chances of experiencing vibrant health throughout our lifetime.

I hope that my discussing how disease develops doesn't make you feel overwhelmed. Through working hard to master our personal environment, each of us has so much control over our health. Finding ways to slow down the personal environmental change that has happened in the last 10,000 years is the only way to ensure that we will live a life free of chronic disease and pass on the best genes we possibly can to our children.

As a result of my conclusions I often get asked why I am obsessed with living forever. Well, I am not obsessed with living forever, and I don't want to live any longer than the maximum lifespan for a human being. However, I want the time I do live to be of high quality. I do not want to spend the last 20 years of my life held back by poor health, unable to do the things I enjoy, which is very common in our older population. I don't fear death; I fear a life in which I am held back from truly living.

Many people do fear death, however. When theorizing as to why humans fear death and show anxiety at its approach, the Nobel prize winning biologist, Elie Metchnikoff, suggested that if we were living full and enjoyable lives that lasted as long as they should, maybe 100 years or so, then we would welcome death as a normal part of life just as we welcome rest after exertion or stop eating once we are satiated. There are many instances of people who experience very advanced age, dying without fear, and on their own terms. Maybe if we were living the length and quality of life that we are evolved to live, death wouldn't be so feared.

As unnecessary as our chronic disease epidemic is, it is also important to note that, as Rene Dubos says, "In reality, complete freedom from disease and from struggle is almost incompatible with living." He is saying that the very process of evolution is based on struggle and those who overcome the struggle win the evolutionary game. But while I acknowledge and accept this, I feel there is much we can do to minimize the unnecessary struggle that has arisen with a chronic disease epidemic stemming from being out of step with our true environment.

In the remainder of this chapter, we survey some of the areas that are most important when thinking about where we can **re**source our lives. As you read through each section I hope you will further see just how much our way of life has changed over the past 10,000 years. This is not intended to be a step-by-step guide but rather an overview of how to approach restoring health (for more in-depth information, refer to the further readings listed in Appendix I). I don't want you to memorize a pre-set list of steps; I want to teach you how to approach life so that you can find ways to improve your health no matter your current environment or history.

Food

If you can make only one change to your current lifestyle, it should be what you put in your mouth every day. As I previously discussed, our diet saw a big change with the Agricultural Revolution as we became more reliant on nutrient-poor crops. However, it has seen an even bigger change within the last 100 years with the excessive processing of those already nutrient-poor crops within the modern food industry. This was so much of a change that I would argue that much of what people in Western countries eat today is not even really food. Food is something that nourishes us. There are 90 essential nutrients—vitamins, minerals, fats, and amino acids (protein)—that our bodies need in order to perform everyday tasks, but many Western "foods" do not get us anywhere close to that quantity. These nutrients are "essential" because the human body cannot synthesize them by itself, and so if we do not get them through our food, then we should not expect our bodies to function properly. I believe that we can get everything we need in the most bioavailable form from eating only animal products as this is what our pre-humans ancestors started eating that allowed us to become modern humans, but I respect those who want to eat plants if they are unprocessed and nutrient dense plants. The healing powers of a nutrient-rich diet are nothing short of miraculous.

To ensure optimal health we need to eat the most nutrient-dense diet we can get our hands on. Getting adequate amounts of those essential nutrients is necessary for the health of our bodies. Looking into how our bodies make energy will show us why. The cells in our bodies have mitochondria—structures that make energy from the food we eat. Just like any energy producing system, waste products are also created through this process. In this case, the by-products of energy creation are carbon dioxide, water, and free radicals (reactive oxygen species). We get rid of the carbon dioxide by breathing, excess water through sweating and breathing, and free radicals are neutralized with antioxidants. Our body makes these antioxidants is we give it the right raw materials, nutrient dense food.

The problem with free radicals it that they oxidize our bodies. Oxidization is the same process that rusts iron when exposed to oxygen in the air for a long time. Yes, free radicals make us rust, so to speak. There are many things that lead to higher numbers of free radicals in our body. If we eat highly refined carbohydrates, our mitochondria will have to work harder to make energy, because you only get 4 kcal of energy from burning a carbohydrate—you get 9 kcal from burning a fat. The mitochondria have to burn more fuel more often when using carbohydrates as fuel, therefore producing more free radicals. Toxicants—which we will discuss more in the next section—also act as free radicals in our bodies. Luckily, to prevent us from oxidizing we have antioxidants that come to the rescue. As I said before, our body makes all the antioxidants it needs but is dependent on us eating the right foods to do so. This mainly consists of a balanced intake of amino acids, or protein. Our bodies evolved to have this nice balance of internally sourced antioxidants that take care of free radicals. However, over the last 10,000 years the amount of processed carbohydrates and toxicants in our lives has steadily increased and the amount quality food we eat has steadily decreased, leading to the "rusting" of humans the world over.

The most impactful change you can make in your diet is to stay away from overly processed foods like sugar, grains, and vegetable oils. These are the most nutrient-poor foods around, and their domination of our food supply has left us severely undernourished and diseased. Instead, we should be seeking out the most nutrient-dense and bioavailable foods we can find: high quality fats, high quality animal products from animals fed their natural diet and in some cases fermented foods, fungal foods and vegetables. Think about it this way: if you were to put watered-down gas or poor quality motor oil in your car then it would not function very well and would come to a halt quicker than if you used the best gas and motor oil. If we don't want our bodies to wear out quicker we need to eat the highest quality foods. If the body lacks raw materials needed to perform metabolic functions then it faces an impossible task. Health is the default state of the body, and your body knows what to do to keep itself from sickness, but we have to do our part by providing it with the best raw materials.

So where do we find the most nutrient-dense food? Nutrient-dense food comes from the natural world, as close as possible to its naturally evolved state. When it comes to food we should ask ourselves what we can get our hands on that is most similar to what our ancient ancestors had available in the wild. Take meat for example. They would have been hunting wild animals. If you have access to wild game meat then that is the best and most nutrient dense meat you could eat. If you don't, then the next best thing would be a domesticated animal that was allowed to eat and live its most natural life. Studies show that grass-fed meats are much more nutrient dense than grain-fed meats, especially the organ meats from grass-fed animals.[3] Fortunately, finding grass-fed or pastured meats is becoming easier and easier. Eating wild or naturally raised animals is very important because when **re**sourcing we are trying to make changes so that we can live as close as we reasonably can to what is natural for us, and therefore we shouldn't be eating animals that live and eat in ways totally unnatural to them.

When we eat grass-fed or pastured meats, we are also supporting the much less toxic—and much more sustainable—practice of grass-fed farming. If enough of us support this type of animal agriculture, it could push the industry away from concentrated animal feeding operations (CAFOs) and lead to a healthier planet. In *Primal Fat Burner,* Nora Gedgaudas shares some staggering statistics about how our current means of food production is destroying our earth. She tells us that 70% of the world's grasslands have been degraded, soil is being depleted 13% faster than it can be rebuilt, and we've lost 75% of the world crop varieties in the last 100 years; additionally, more than a billion people don't have fresh drinking water, while 80% of the world's freshwater is being used for industrial agriculture. When you think about agriculture as it pertains to natural ecology, it is no surprise that we are in this situation. In the natural world we see diversity; every plant and animal plays a role in sustaining life within an ecosystem. Every plant takes different nutrients from the soil so as not to deplete the soil of any certain set of nutrients, plants keep each other in check through competing for space, and animals help to spread seeds and fertilize soil so that it can continue to support plant life. When we started agriculture 10,000 years ago we completely defied this process. We cleared land of all diversity, kept animals off that land, and planted the same crop year after year until the soil was so dead it could not support crops any longer. It is even a common theory among scientists—like Jared Diamond in his book, *Collapse*—that many previous civilizations have fallen as a result of crop failure, or were torn apart by wars due to scarcity of food or resources.

Whether it's how we grow crops or raise animals, our modern food system is not sustainable. Many people chose to revert to extreme diets like veganism in order to boycott one practice or another within this system. But in this case the best way to combat these practices, while also achieving health, is not an extreme diet. Eating animals is not what is contributing to these issues; it's the way we choose to raise these animals. The solution is to raise animals in a way that is natural for them, sustainable for the environment, and will result in a healthier version of ourselves. The answer is grass feeding or pasture raising our animals. I highly recommend looking into the Savory Institute to learn about how this type of farming is the most sustainable way to provide us with high quality meat and how it will actually restore life to our land. To help you find sources of grass-fed or pastured meat near you go to eatwild.com.

As far as how to sustainably eat plant food, our ancestors would have eaten wild plants directly out of the woods and only when high quality animal food was not available. If you can learn to forage safely and use that as a source for food then that would be a very nutrient dense and sustainable option. However, I realize that for most people that is not a realistic plan, and if all 7 billion people on the planet started foraging, that wouldn't be very sustainable either. So if you're going to eat much plant food the next best thing would be local organic produce. Organic merely means that a farmer met the standards of growing food that they needed to in order to legally label their food organic. Therefore, organic does not mean that it is free of all toxins. The process is not perfect, and the politics are just as complicated as anything else. However, upon testing, organic food has far fewer harmful chemicals, is much more nutrient dense,[4] and since organic food is not allowed to be GMO, it is a clear vote against that huge genetic food experiment. It makes sense when you think about it. Just like in humans, nutrients are what help plants defend themselves. If we use lots of herbicides and pesticides to create an environment with few natural threats to the plant, then not only are we contaminating the plant and environment but we are making it so that the plant doesn't work hard to acquire the nutrients it would have needed to survive. The result is scarcer nutrients. Further, the herbicide glyphosate, which is widely sprayed on GMO crops, destroys the mineral content of the soil, making it impossible for plants to get enough minerals. By choosing organic you are voting for a more natural world, and if enough of us make that choice then maybe we can stop the pollution of our farmlands and halt the production of genetically modified crops—all while improving our health.

It is also important to eat as local as possible. The moment a food is picked from a plant or harvested from an animal it slowly starts losing nutrients, so the sooner we eat it the better chance we have of absorbing all the nutrition that the food has to offer us. Also, local food travels less distance, and therefore depletes fewer of our natural resources. Going to a farmers market and buying directly from the farmers—who can even tell you about their precise farming practices—is a great way to increase nutrient content in your food and decrease the cost of resources it takes to get it to you.

Before we leave the topic of plants we have to talk a little about anti-nutrients. Remember when I was talking about a proper ecosystem where the animals help spread plant seeds by eating and pooping them out? That works well for some plants and their seeds, but other plants don't like animals, including humans, to eat their seeds because they get destroyed in our digestive tracts. These plants have evolved defense mechanisms to discourage animals from eating them. Some examples of anti-nutrients are lectins (found in grains and some vegetables), phytic acid (found in legumes), oxalates (found in some greens), and tannins (found in many teas). These are just some of the types of anti-nutrients and some of the places they are found. Anti-nutrients can wreak havoc on the body, especially its immune system. Foods high in anti-nutrients were generally not available to our hunter-gatherer ancestors and eliminating anti-nutrients can be a very useful part of any health-achieving strategy. For some people this could mean removing all plant toxins by removing all plants from their diet.

Perhaps even more important than eating local and organic and avoiding anti-nutrients is acknowledging that our ancient ancestors ate a lot of fat, a highly sought after nutrient. Eating a high fat diet from healthy, wild animals or fat-dense plants is what allowed our brains to grow as big as they did and ultimately, along with the development of weapons and hunting strategies, what enabled some of our ancestors to migrate out of Africa and live in the many different climates of the world. When our ancestors killed and ate a wild animal it was a huge trove of nutrients. They didn't just eat the meat; they ate the organs and the bone marrow, which are much more nutrient dense than the meat alone. It turns out that the low fat craze of the last half century is one of the worst ideas modern humans have had. Low fat diets have been starving our brains and destroying our energy-making mitochondria. Fat is also what allows us to utilize the fat-soluble vitamins A, D, E, and K that are critical to our health. The drop in levels of these nutrients due to low fat diets has been a main contributor to our chronic disease epidemic. When we increase the amount of high quality fat from healthy animals humans thrive and their chances of getting disease is significantly reduced. We need fat, and our body loves it.

Fat does not make us fat either. One of the reasons that people think that it does is because in the English language the word "fat" is used for dietary fat as well as body fat, creating a misconception that eating fat will make you fat. In many other languages they are much more specific when talking about fat. For example, in Hungarian the word for dietary fat is "zsir," and the word to describe someone as overweight is "kövér," and the words are not interchangeable. It turns out that the amount of calories we eat has very little effect on whether or not we gain weight. For the majority of people, our bodies put on weight when we eat too many empty carbohydrates (processed wheat, corn, sugar, and soy), have an imbalance in our gut bacteria (excess antibiotics), or have too many toxins stored in our body. By increasing the amount of high quality fats in our diet we create a much more energy efficient fat-burning machine that is more effective at doing everything from rocket science to weight lifting to soccer moming. In case you were wondering, yes, I am telling you that you can eat grass-fed butter, pastured eggs, grass-fed steak and liver, and pastured bacon—and they are very healthy for you!

"Wait," you may be thinking, "What about heart disease?" It also turns out that the cause of heart disease is not fat or cholesterol. A 2014 review of 72 studies on dietary fat and cholesterol done in eighteen countries showed absolutely no correlation between dietary fat and heart disease.[5] Poor cholesterol was framed. The real cause of heart disease is twofold. The first cause is the increase in the amount of stress and the dysfunctional response to stress that we have in society these days. This leads to an imbalance of the sympathetic and parasympathetic nervous systems that can send us down the road to a heart attack.[6]The second factor is the rise in inflammation brought on by the excessive consumption of processed grains, sugar, and vegetable oils. These foods can damage the lining of the artery walls, causing cholesterol to try and repair them—which puts it at the scene of the crime, so to speak, and is why it has been framed. We have been completely misled when it comes to heart disease. All this is proven when people with lots of high quality fat in their diets experience greater health and less heart disease than those without it[7] and is further proven because, despite the low fat craze of the last half century, when we replaced saturated fats with vegetable oils, heart disease continued to rise. There is even research showing that people with higher cholesterol levels live longer![8]

Another form of "food" I'd like to spend some time on is supplements. The two main problems with most supplements are that they are synthetic nutrients and they are isolated. We evolved to eat whole, natural foods that provide many nutrients packaged together. Those nutrients work synergistically to nourish our body. We cannot take a nutrient out of a food (or create it in a lab) and expect it to do the same thing in the body as it would if it came naturally in the food. The supplement industry has also become just as profit driven as the pharmaceutical industry. Many brands are making low quality products and charging tons of money for them. Trying to eat an okay diet and then supplementing with synthetic nutrients is not a good path to health. Further, at Consumer Wellness Center Labs they have been randomly testing supplements off the shelf and have found many of them are highly contaminated with heavy metals and/or have very little amounts of the products they claim to have.

However, there are times when pharmaceutical doses of certain isolated vitamin and mineral supplements can be used to treat certain disease processes. For example, intravenous vitamin C for cancer has shown huge promise.[9] There are also many food grade supplements that are very worth taking and can really help us in our quest to get enough nutrition amongst the rapidly dropping nutrient content of our food supply. I heard a good argument for supplements on a podcast one time (admittedly I've lost the source). It was argued that if we should get all our nutrients from nature, then everything else we come in contact with should be from nature as well. From this perspective the only toxicants we should be exposed to are those naturally occurring in nature, yet in today's world we are overwhelmed with unnatural toxicants daily. Since we have this unnatural exposure, and the nutrients in our bodies are the number one defense against these toxicants, then high quality food grade supplements can be very useful in our battle against toxicants. When looking for good supplements, we should stick to smaller companies where the owner is the one who does most of the promoting. It is good to see someone selling their products because they are passionate about health and have priorities other than just making a profit. It is also a good idea to buy from companies who have a third party verification certification so that we can be confident we are getting what is promised.

Another useful perspective on food is to realize that we live in a binary world where it is popular to demonize some things and glorify others; everything either tends to be labeled good or bad. As a society, we go through cycles of making certain foods or nutrients good or bad all the time. While there are some foods that are just not compatible with health in humans, in reality we should not label a food as good or bad. We should look at where the food came from and how it was grown or raised. Diary is a good example. Most of the dairy in the grocery stores comes from cows that are very unhealthy due to the fact that they are fed an unnatural diet, pumped full of antibiotics and hormones, and given terrible living conditions. On top of that, the milk that they do produce is pasteurized and homogenized, destroying anything good that was left. People go back and forth saying we should drink milk or we shouldn't, but what really matters is how that milk in the store got there and what happened to it on the journey. While it is curious that we are the only mammal that drinks milk into adulthood and the only mammal that drinks another mammal's milk, dairy can be a very nutrient dense food, and some forms of dairy can be very important in healing certain imbalances in the body. So the last lesson on food is not to ask if a food is good or bad, but to ask how that food's journey affected the final product. Did it leave it nutrient poor and damaged or nutrient dense and whole? By learning these things about your food you will never have to wonder if what you are eating is feeding disease or fighting it.

I understand that processing all this and trying to rearrange your diet to fit all these requirements can be overwhelming at first. One of the best ways to approach it is to make an effort to increase the nutrient quality of your food by eating in a way that has less impact on the planet. We can do this by getting more connected with where food comes from. Don't focus so much on which food has which nutrients—just eat nutrient dense, bioavailable foods and investigate where the food came from and how it was grown or raised. The more natural the process of growing or raising the food, the more nutrient dense it will be. There are many ways to do this. As I mentioned before, one way is to find the nearest farmers' market. Another way to get connected with food is to produce some of your own. If you want to include plants, you can grow an herb garden in the window of your kitchen and a vegetable garden in the backyard. If you have the space, you can get a couple of chickens for eggs. Getting more in touch with food connects you with the environment in ways that are hard for people living in the modern world to see otherwise. It may also give you a sense of satisfaction and provide fun and educational activities for the kids.

I hope that the above approach to food will guide you in making better decisions for your diet, regardless of a specific situation. If you find you don't know where to begin, my recommendation is to start by eliminating processed foods such as sugar, grains, and vegetable oils and making sure you get plenty of healthy, fat-filled foods from animals as often as you can. Next, if you want to eat plants, add wild plants to your diet, if you have access to them. If you don't, the next best option is organic and local produce. Finally, avoid the anti-nutrients and "low fat" recommendations, as discussed above, and do your homework on supplements.

For more complete guides that give you varying opinions on eating the cleanest, most unaltered nutrient dense diet, I recommend the books, *Deep Nutrition* by Cate Shanahan, MD, *The Bulletproof Diet* by Dave Asprey, *The Plant Paradox* by Steven Gundry, and *Nourishing Traditions* by Sally Fallon.

Toxicants

The second most important thing to consider about your personal environment is how many toxicants you come into contact with on a daily basis. Learning how to reduce your exposure to the unending amount of toxicants in our world is critical when trying to achieve health. Second to food, this is the aspect of our environment that has changed the most drastically, especially in the last 200 years. I will warn you here, once you start learning all the sources of toxicants in the world today you can go crazy trying to avoid them all. It is near impossible to avoid them all, and I don't recommend trying—just realize that it is important to make an effort to avoid as many as you can. The good news is that the best thing you can do to protect yourself against them is what we just discussed: eat nutrient dense, bioavailable food. Still, even if you do eat a perfect diet, you will find that your body will also thank you for avoiding as many toxicants as possible.

Toxicants have gotten so out of hand because, through processes like chemical engineering, we have taken the naturally occurring molecules and compounds of our world and rearranged them in ways that the body has never seen before. While doing this has created advancements in how we live, it is one major example of how humans may have become too smart for our own good. The massive influx of unnatural chemicals and toxicants into our world is one of the major drivers of change in personal environment. If manmade toxic compounds synthesized by scientists had naturally formed in the environment, they would have done so hand-in-hand with evolution, allowing living things to adapt. But when you unleash millions of toxic chemicals within a short period of time, life is going to struggle to deal with that change. Personally, I think it is amazing that our bodies are able to detoxify them at all given that they appeared on the scene so quickly and there is no way we have had time to evolve to be better detoxifiers.

Not all toxicants are the same and there are many different toxicants that surround us. They fall into two groups, non-persistent and persistent. The non-persistent ones are relatively easy for our bodies to get rid of, but that is not the case for the persistent ones. When non-persistent toxicants cycle through our detoxification organs (mainly liver and kidneys) they are easily handled as long as we have adequate nutrition. This is not to say that we should not worry about the non-persistent toxicants, as constant exposure can negatively affect our bodies. On the other hand, detoxification organs are not always able to detoxify persistent toxicants. To get rid of them we have to make sure we have adequate amounts of various nutrients in our body, and even with those nutrients, persistent toxicants are stubborn. As we have discussed, the average American is starving their body of nutrients while unknowingly increasing their toxicant exposure. As a result, the body ends up having to store many toxicants in tissues for lack of a better option.

Many toxicants are fat-soluble and the body ends up storing them in excess body fat or fatty tissues like the brain or the breast. This can lead to things like neurodegenerative diseases[10] and breast cancer.[11] It can also make weight loss much harder because the body can't afford to mobilize stored fat. Burning this fat would also release stored toxicants that overwhelm the liver because it rarely has the nutrients it needs to handle them, which is why the toxicants got stored in the first place. Since the liver runs our metabolism, when it becomes overwhelmed this can severely slow metabolism and halt weight loss in its tracts. This is evident when we see people working for hours in the gym with no results and more evident when the only thing I do with a health-coaching client is a personal environment detoxification protocol and they start losing weight.

There are two phases of detoxification in your liver and a third phase which is excreting the toxic waste. It is not necessary to get into the ins and outs of these phases here, just know that when phase one happens the toxicant is transformed into something more toxic and oxidative—more rust causing. The body relies on phase two to immediately pick it up and transform it into something that the body can excrete through the bowels, kidneys, or sweat. If these phases are not balanced we end up with a traffic jam of more damaging toxic intermediates in the liver. Guess what ensures that the system stays balanced? Adequate nutrients. A nutrient dense diet is essential for protecting against toxicants.

If you are sitting there thinking that you may not come into contact with that many toxicants, think again. They are everywhere. Toxicants are found on produce, in meat products, in tap water, in cosmetics, in cleaning supplies and laundry detergent, in vaccines, in the air we breathe, on cookware, in anything plastic, in many supplements, in water-damaged buildings, on furniture and clothes, and in your dental fillings. Even the wrong kind of light or electromagnetic energy can be a toxicant, which we'll discuss more in later sections. Avoiding as many sources of toxicants as possible and safeguarding ourselves against the ones we do come in contact with is an extremely important part of living a life closer to the one we evolved in for millions of years. It is not hard to imagine that our ancient environment had far fewer toxicants floating around.

How avoiding toxicants will help save our planet, and therefore us, is likely obvious, but a popular example is the amount of plastic that ends up in the ocean. It has been reported that the amount of plastic waste in the ocean has affected at least 267 species worldwide, including 86% of all sea turtle species, 44% of all seabird species and 43% of all marine mammal species. The impacts include fatalities as a result of ingestion, starvation, suffocation, infection, drowning, and entanglement.[12] Remember, we are part of the natural world and things that have a negative effect on it have a negative effect on us as well. Plastics are hormone disruptors, and as mentioned before, have been linked to diseases like breast cancer in women[11] and low testosterone in men.[13]

Common plasticizers like Bisphenol A (BPA) are very common. We are exposed to them any time we drink from plastic bottles, use plastic storage containers, or grab our receipts from our last purchase. Even plastics that are "BPA free" contain other plasticizers that are no less harmful. As consumers, if we start showing companies that we want products that are free of substances not compatible with our bodies then they will be forced to make their products cleaner in order to stay in business. This will also prevent many toxicants from being pumped into our personal and global environments and therefore tilt our world a little bit back in the direction of what it used to look like prior to 10,000 years ago.

It is important to realize that no matter how hard we try we will never avoid all the toxicants we are exposed to. The key is to avoid the ones you have control over and not stress about the ones you don't. One of the easiest ways to reduce much of our toxicant exposure is by filtering our air and water. By putting quality air filters in the places we spend our most time—home and work—we take big leaps in reducing our exposure. I like the air filters made by Air Oasis and Air Doctor and we will discuss water in more detail in the next section. For a complete guide to all the exposures of toxicants in our world you can read Dr. Walter Crinnion's book, *Clean, Green, and Lean*. I suggest reading one chapter at a time to implement toxicant avoidance strategies slowly so you don't overwhelm yourself or your family with all the changes.

Water

I don't have to tell you how important water is to maintaining the health of our bodies; we all know it is essential for life. Unfortunately, all water is not created equal....well, it was created equal and then humans happened. The water that comes out of our tap is pretty dead; it is overly recycled, mineral poor, and full of toxicants. This happens purposefully in some cases, like the government adding neurotoxic fluoride to the drinking water,[14] but also unintentionally from people flushing all kinds of things down the toilet, like unused medications or the toxicants found in their own waste. Unfortunately, the current filtration of our municipal water—while it does make the water "safe" to drink—does not account for many of the toxicants that end up in our water system, and they end up getting put right back into our tap water.

If you think that bottled water will save you from tap water then you are in for a rude awakening. Most bottled waters are nothing more than glorified tap water. Plus, they are wrapped in toxic plastic that seeps into the water and ultimately ends up polluting our bodies and our planet. As mentioned in the toxicant section, plastic is a toxicant that is having a large effect on our hormones as it can mimic estrogen in the body.[15] Obviously, if it is the only option available, especially in an emergency situation, it can keep people alive. But if we are looking for vibrant health we need to find a different source of water.

Our ancient ancestors would have found water free flowing, mineral-rich, and filtered by the earth. In those days it was safe to drink water flowing in a river or stream. These days we would be taking a risk doing that. However, naturally flowing springs produce water that maintains its health-promoting qualities. To make our personal environment the most like that of our pre-agriculture ancestors, we should find a clean spring and collect water from it. You can go to www.findaspring.com and locate the spring nearest you. I recommend reading up on the spring you plan to use and maybe even testing the water before you start to drink it.

If that doesn't sound like something you would be able to do, then you need to look at filtering your water. Filtered water may not be as mineral-rich as we would like but at least it will be free of all the toxicants swimming around in our tap water. However, all water filters are not created equal. Finding one that is the most effective at getting rid of the wide range of toxicants in your water is essential. For a smaller counter top filter I recommend the Aquatru brand (electric) and for a larger filter I recommend Big Berkey (gravity filter). These are the best but if all you can afford is a pitcher filter then it is better than nothing; it will at least reduce the amount of fluoride and chlorine you drink.

There are some bottled waters that are suitable to drink but they are typically the expensive natural mineral spring waters. One of the ones I often get is San Pellegrino. It is distributed by a corporation that has some sketchy business practices, but the water itself is good and has a high amount of sulfates. Sulfates are very useful in helping our livers get rid of toxicants. I also like it because you can get it in glass bottles, which helps us decrease the amount of plastic pumped into our bodies and the environment. I know, I know, by supporting a corporation that is not optimal then we are not quite voting with our dollar to change the world and ensure the survival of the species, but sometimes none of the choices presented to us are perfect. If we are collecting our water from a spring or filtering it and if we are pushing for a more advanced filtration process for municipal water then we are making some change. We will likely have to settle for adequate bottled waters on occasion.

Maybe one day we can even get the government to structure the municipal water supply. What is structured water you may ask? There is more to water than meets the eye. Structuring water is an approach that you can take if you really want to achieve the highest level of health from the water you drink. Dr. Gerald Pollack at the University of Washington has discovered that water is not the simple liquid we thought it was, and that it doesn't always demonstrate the properties of a liquid. He has shown that water, when put under certain conditions, has a fourth phase that happens between solid and liquid. Your body prefers the water that is able to get into this structured phase and actually works to make this happen. It is becoming evident through what Pollack is learning in his lab that water has much more to do with a healthy body than just hydration, and that getting or building structured water in your body is an important aspect of health.

Returning to the theme of moving toward a life similar to our ancient ancestors, it turns out that one of the ways that we can get structured water is by collecting it from a natural spring. Due to high pressures when the water is deep underground it becomes structured. Another way that water can become structured is by exposure to infrared light. We could do this in our body by getting adequate sun exposure without burning, or we could use infrared saunas. Infrared saunas conveniently help with our toxicant problem as well because they help us sweat—a natural detoxifier—and the light also penetrates the skin to pull out those persistent toxicants. Yet another way to get structured water is by vortexing the water. We can do this by getting a vortex device for our homes. Interestingly, when we look at blood going through the heart, the shape of the heart chambers actually vortexes the blood as it moves through them.[16] The human body is so complex and fascinating.

As far as what structured water can do for our planet, it turns out that when a tube made with a substance that has hydrophilic properties is placed in structured water, the water begins to flow through the tube with no outside force. The physics of how this works is beautifully explained in Dr. Pollack's' book. This may help explain how blood can flow from the feet back up to the heart, but it is also important because currently we use all kinds of natural resources to create energy that we can use to get water to flow, like pumping water to a house or to water fields. But the properties of structured water show us that all we need to do is create the right conditions for water to flow on its own. If we focused research and development on this revolutionary characteristic of water, we could harness this "work-creating" property and spare the use of so many natural resources.

For more information on the unknown properties of water you can get Dr. Pollack's book, *The Fourth Phase of Water*.

Gut Health

If there is one thing that can show us how connected we are to the grand ecosystem that is our planet, it is the microbiome— the ecosystem we have inside our own bodies. The bacteria that live in and on us make up our microbiome and the digestive system houses a large portion of it. I will let Rene Dubos, who we have heard from before in this book, open up this section by illustrating the importance of ecosystem balance:

The difficulties that may follow antibacterial therapy are in fact similar in essence to those encountered in any attempt to control predators in nature. Because so many leopards have been killed in Africa there is now a plague of baboons which destroy the crops in certain areas. [...] On the Kaibab Plateau extermination of the wolves and mountain lions has proved unfavorable in the long run to the deer by allowing them to multiply excessively and overgraze their feeding areas. Whether the method of treatment affects the animal predators in the wilderness or the bacteria in the gut, it is always risky to tamper with the natural balance of forces in nature.

It is vitally important to maintain a diverse ecosystem of microbes in your body. Your digestive system is basically an external environment inside your body, extending from mouth to anus. It is sealed off to the outside word and filled with microorganisms. This microbiome is important because it helps us digest our food, aids in regulation of the immune system, and sends signals to our brain about what may be going on in our external environment. Research even shows that our gut sends more signals to our brain than our brain sends to our gut.[17] As Dubos illustrated, ecosystems are linked, and one aspect of an ecosystem cannot change without affecting the others. You can imagine that the major changes in our way of life have had a drastic impact on the ecosystem that is the human body.

Earlier in this chapter we discussed some things that can contribute to gut microbiome imbalances, such as cesarean birth, not being breast fed, and unneeded courses of antibiotics. These are huge contributors to the epidemic of gut issues that range from indigestion to Crohn's Disease. Some other contributors are, you guessed it, poor diet, but also the herbicide glyphosate (thanks, Monsanto*), which we are exposed to in greater amounts when eating a diet that is not organic. Are you starting to see just how important a nutrient-rich organic diet is? When it comes to gut health a good diet is important because what we eat can affect the ratios of bacterium. A balance of bacteria in our gut is important in the same sense that the balance of various species in a natural ecosystem is important, as Dubos illustrated above. There will always be "bad" bacteria in our gut, but we want more of the "good" kind that we have a symbiotic relationship with to hold the "bad" in check. Symbiotic means that both parties benefit from the interaction. We provide the bacteria a place to live and reproduce and they hold the "bad" bacteria in check as well as help us with digestion and signal our bodies to perform certain tasks. Having certain ratios of bacteria in your gut can even trigger your body to either lose or gain weight.[18]

The ratio of gut bacteria is important because your gut is like a parking lot in that there are only so many spaces. Going back to the scenario discussed early in this chapter, if a human is a cesarean birth, is not breast fed, takes many doses of unnecessary antibiotics, and eats a processed food diet, then they are bound to end up with all their parking spaces taken up by "bad" bacteria. These "bad" bacteria feed off of processed grains and sugars, and if you eat a diet high in these foods you just solidify the "bad" bacteria's hold on those parking spaces. Conversely, if we eat a nutrient rich, whole food diet then we create an environment that the "bad" bacteria don't like and we feed the "good" bacteria, allowing them to kick the "bad" out.

Unfortunately, not all the different strains of gut bacteria can be restored once they are lost. It is possible for one dose of antibiotics to cause a strain of bacteria to go extinct within our microbiome and, depending on the strain that was lost, we may never get it back. Normally, we have hundreds of different species of bacteria in our digestive tract. One course of antibiotics can have major impacts on that diversity, and since we don't necessarily have surefire ways of restoring all that diversity yet, it is urgent that you start healing your gut and protecting that symbiotic bacteria as soon as possible by avoiding toxins that kill those microbes and eating a diet that feeds them. There is research suggesting that the quantity of good bacteria in your gut is not nearly as important as the diversity of strains in our microbiome,[19] and diversity in gut health has a direct correlation to better health outcomes.

Nothing screams, "I'm living like our ancient ancestors!" more than a healthy microbiome. I say this because when you are in the natural world, eating natural food, drinking natural water, and in contact with the earth, then creating a healthy microbiome is unavoidable.[20] However, since our drastic lifestyle changes—especially since the germ theory of disease showed up—we have been living in a germophobic world, depriving our bodies of this life-giving bacteria. Back in the day, we were in continual contact with the earth. We were exposed to animals that we killed and food that was sometimes a little old and fermented, and we were in contact with each other. A diversity of bacteria abounded at these points of contact. Don't get me wrong, some bacteria and viruses are not good for us, but those bacteria did not evolve to be problematic for humans or animals until we started living in large groups in close proximity to each other and domesticated animals, and they would not affect us nearly as much if our microbial diversity was intact. Since bacteria and viruses can reproduce quickly, some in less than an hour, the ones that cause infectious disease evolved very quickly once we started living in large groups, where the bacteria could find a new host quickly if it killed the first. They have even taken advantage of when our immune system fights them off in a process we know as coughing, sneezing, and having a runny nose. These actions on our part help them find a new host by letting us do the work of spreading them out.

There is a fine line between getting as many germs as possible without contracting the infectious ones, but we are going about avoiding the latter in the wrong ways. It may seem counterintuitive, but antibacterial soap and hand sanitizer is actually increasing our likelihood of contracting an infectious disease by creating antibiotic resistant bacteria[21] and decreasing our microbial diversity. Ironically, you need *more* bacteria (of the good variety!) in order to be more resilient to the infectious ones. It is estimated that 70-80% of our immune system is in our gut,[22] and if we have a healthy diversity of gut bacteria and a healthy gut lining, our immune system is better able to do its job. By over-sanitizing everything we are weakening our immune system, leaving us more susceptible to infectious disease.

The balance of bacteria is not the only important aspect of gut health; we also have to pay attention to the structural component of our digestive system. Many of us have heard the term leaky gut, as it has become a buzz word in the health world. Understanding leaky gut can help us appreciate the importance of gut health. Leaky gut is when we develop tiny holes in the digestive tube that runs from the mouth to the anus. Normally, that tube is sealed off from the body's other systems. When the tube has holes in it—which can happen from not being breast fed, taking antibiotics, ingesting the pesticide glyphosate, or inflammation from imbalances in bacteria—then the contents of the gut can "leak" into the blood stream and cause all kinds of problems. Portions of undigested food, the microbiome, toxicants, and whatever else might be in the gut can end up in places they are not supposed to be. The constant leaking causes the body's immune system to be on high alert all the time, creating an overactive immune system.

This overactive state can lead to health complications such as allergies, food intolerances, and autoimmune disorders.

Recently, the gut has been shown to have an extensive relationship with the brain. Some neurologists, including Dr. David Perlmutter, have even treated various neurological conditions through gut-healing protocols. The results are nothing short of amazing. Conditions that are supposedly neurological—like depression and dementia—are treated through the gut, yielding outcomes that are unheard of in Western medicine. This is just one example of how interconnected the systems of the body are, and it illustrates how our healthcare system's approach to treating systems in isolation will never work. By treating only the organ or organ system that is presenting with symptoms, we are missing that often times those symptoms are presenting because of dysfunction in another part of the body. Through my clinical experience I can say that paying attention to gut health is not just important for digestion, it is critical in just about all disease processes.

Hopefully, I have convinced you of the importance of gut health, but how do we achieve it? In order to ensure proper gut health, we need to—you've got it—get back in touch with nature. Go for a barefoot walk in the park or a hike in the woods and soak up nature's bacteria. Planting a garden will not only provide you with nutrient-dense food without causing the destruction of our earth, it will also get you in touch with the earth's bacteria. Eat fermented foods like sauerkraut, kim chi, and kefir to introduce some good bacteria into your personal ecosystem. Lastly, avoid antibiotics unless you have a life-threatening infection, and eat foods—like root vegetables and bone broth—that promote a healthy balance of bacteria.

Not only do the bacteria of the world play an important role for us, they are critical in the health of the ecosystem of our entire planet. Just like the change in lifestyle of 10,000 years ago gradually had a negative effect on our personal ecosystem, it has had a negative effect on the global ecosystem as well. The spraying of our crops with herbicides, pesticides, and fertilizers is destroying the bacterial ecosystem of the soil that our food grows in.[23] It has been reported that 12 million hectares of land, an area the size of Benin, are lost every year and US $42 billion in income is lost every year from desertification and land degradation.[24] What happens when our land is so dead that it can no longer grow our food? To help prevent us from getting to this point I think that if we, as consumers, start demanding nutrient-rich organic food, it will drive changes in the way the industry produces our food and therefore begin to restore life to our soils. Again, the Savory Institute is doing great work in restoring life to our soil, and I highly recommend learning from what they do.

Believe it or not, working hard to achieve gut health may also be critically important for creating a more cooperative and peaceful world among humans. This is illustrated by two recent research studies. In the first study researchers were able to reduce risk-taking behavior in mice by giving them products that created a healthier ratio of gut microbes.[25] Another study showed that feeding women a fermented milk product rich in probiotics modulated brain activity.[26] In this case they found that they were able to reduce the emotional response to negative stimuli in women who ate the probiotic product. Achieving gut health could help us achieve the healthy, peaceful mind necessary to allow us to come together and solve many big world issues.

Using strategies I have suggested can upgrade your gut and lead to a healthier you. However, if your gut is really imbalanced you may require the guidance of a knowledgeable healthcare practitioner. We will talk about how to find one of those in a future section. There is also the microbiome testing company called

Viome that provides very educational and practical information for achieving individualized gut health. For more information about the amazing gut ecosystem and how to maintain a healthy microbiome as well as the role of microbes in our world, check out the book, *The Skinny Gut Diet* by Brenda Watson, *Brain Maker* by David Perlmutter, MD, and *I Contain Multitudes* by Ed Yong.

*Regarding Monsanto: When you look at a company that has the track record of making chemicals like Agent Orange and DDT—two things proven to have detrimental effects on health—you would think that it would be time to thoroughly test every single product that came out of that company before exposing the general public to it.

Movement

It is likely pretty obvious how much our physical activity has changed in recent history. For millions of years humans and our ancestors spent all day moving their bodies in order to hunt or find food, escape danger, and protect their young. Now most people work at jobs where they are sedentary and then go to the store to buy processed foods. Some people try to make up for that sedentary lifestyle by cramming an hour of intense exercise at the gym into their day, but even that is very different from the way our ancestors used to move. The complete change in how we acquire the necessities of survival has altered our movement patterns in ways that are detrimental to our health.

Whether you believe it's by design or by evolution, we are meant to move more that we do. We evolved to move efficiently in the natural environment. For our ancestors, those who weren't able to do so likely didn't make it. Therefore, evolution selected the best movers—not just of our species, but of every species. Natural selection made a large percentage of our bodies into skeletal muscle that we used to use extensively every day. Therefore, if we want to slow the personal environmental changes that are causing us so much disease then we too need to use our muscles extensively every day.

The good news is that you won't have to spend hours at the gym to match a more ancestral lifestyle. Let's take a look at what an ancestral movement pattern would have looked like. We may never know for sure how much exercise our ancestors got, but one unwritten law of the natural world is that you should conserve energy whenever you can and only use it when the chances are high that it will be worth the effort. Those high pay-off times would have been to hunt a probable kill, escape a threat, or protect your offspring (and genetic line). These situations would have created times when intense exercise was necessary. So while moderate movement of our body would have happened daily, intense exercise may not have been an everyday thing.

As a matter of fact, research is now suggesting that long bouts of intense exercise are not that good for us. It leads to excess inflammation, cardiovascular damage, and oxidative stress (rust)[27] and tends to wear down parts of the body (knees and hips). When it comes to exercise it is more important to make sure the movements we are doing are effective—meaning we are getting the most out of the movement in a reasonable amount of time—and efficient, meaning we are not causing ourselves harm through excess inflammation and structural damage. It is less important to focus on mileage, heart rate, or quantity of time. By doing functional movements we can ensure that we are getting the most effective and efficient movement possible. However, even if it is functional movement, it is important that there is not an imbalance between periods of heavy movement, like intense gym sessions, and then no movement, like me sitting here for hours writing a book.

Functional movement means that you are moving your body in ways that the body is adapted to move. Our muscles have evolved to work in a synergistic manner, meaning it is extremely rare that one muscle or group of muscles acts alone. If I was gathering some food out in the woods and a cougar jumped out and tried to kill me, I wouldn't fire one muscle at a time to try and get away. Flexing your leg up, and then extending your lower leg out, and then activating your glutes to put your foot down all in individual movements would likely yield poor results in this situation. Instead, all of my muscles would be working together at the same time. From the large muscles of my legs to the tiny ciliary muscles in my eyes, they all would be put to use to give me a chance to escape. This means that to mimic how we would move in our natural environment, we need to move our bodies in ways that reinforce natural, complex movements.

An example of the exact opposite of natural movement is a bicep curl. Here we are training our brain to activate only one set of muscles—the muscles that flex the forearm toward our shoulder. Exercises like biceps curls or leg curls create imbalance in the way our brain creates movement, not only leaving us at a disadvantage when being chased by cougars, but also making us more prone to injury in the world we live in today. This is because, aside from movement, our muscles act as shock absorbers to our joints. Our muscles not only cause movement, they protect us when we make movements that put us at risk of injury. Weakness of stabilization muscles and poor functional movement contribute to these types of injuries, and they are very common in our society.

As a chiropractor I see many back injuries, and I will say that most back injuries are due to muscle imbalances from a lack of functional movement or overuse of a muscle doing non-functional movements. For example, some of the main protectors of the lower spine are the four different sets of abdominal muscles that we all have. Unfortunately, many people don't spend much time making sure their abs are strong enough to support their lower back. Even those who do lots of weight training usually focus on the abs in the front (rectus abdominus, or the "six pack") and ignore the abs that wrap all the way around to the low back (the transverse and obliques). A sudden, unguarded movement is the most common mechanism of injury I hear of for the low back injury called a herniated disc. People say they got up to answer the phone, they stepped off a curb wrong, or they reacted to a toddler about to do something dangerous. If your core muscles are not trained, or are improperly trained, then they do not activate in time or in the right way to protect the structures of your low back from injury as you make these quick movements. Functional training of the core, working in synergy with the rest of your muscles, is essential for injury prevention.

With a brilliant analogy to food, which we have already discussed, Katy Bowman captures functional movement perfectly:

> As with food, we're missing wisdom when it comes to movement. The bulk of the exercises we're told to do are human-made. They contain elements of nature—an elbow bend, an extended hip, an arched back—but they are blended with other motions, specifically manufactured equipment, a special building, required footwear, and the right outfit. Our exercises are just like processed food. They're not necessarily the most nutritious; they're just the easiest for us to produce within our sedentary lifestyle. They're all that we know to eat because we come from a sedentary culture where there's hardly anyone left to hand down the practice of movement.

While I completely agree with Katy, let me clarify that weight training, or other kinds of strength and resistance exercises, are great additions to an exercise routine. We just need to be sure that we are implementing functional movements. In general, functional exercises involve moving more than one joint and more than one set of muscles. So instead of that bicep curl you can try doing pull-ups or chin-ups—with support, if needed. Pulling up on a bar looks a lot more like something a human in the wild would do, such as when climbing a tree. Try and make your workout movements in the gym as much like the running, jumping, squatting, swimming, climbing, and crawling that our wild ancestors would have been doing. Obviously, this can start with strength training in the gym but it should eventually evolve to more complex natural movements. Further, our ancestors would not have exercised with intensity any longer than they had to. Remember, conserving energy could have been the difference between life and death back then. Short periods of intense exercise—termed "burst training"— would likely be most similar to what our ancestors did to chase food, flea from predators, and protect offspring. To be clear, I do not think exercises such as long, intense runs lasting more than 20-30 minutes are good for us; they just create more inflammation and wear and tear in our bodies.

Even better than going to the gym, the most beneficial form of movement is one that takes you through your natural environment. My favorite form of exercise is hiking for camping. Not only does it give me exercise that can improve balance, stamina, and strength, it also puts me in contact with the earth, and gives my body all the signals that it is home, which let it know to relax (more about this in the section on stress). In her book, *Movement Matters,* Katy Bowman shows us how important it is to move in the natural world. She says that chronic diseases are caused "by our attempt to live outside of nature, inside walls that limit how far we can see, chairs that prevent our hips and knees from bending all the way to get us to the floor, and thermostats that keep our body temperature at a constant, with no physiological work involved." She suggests that we can continue to sit unmoving in our homes and then try to boost the intensity of our one hour of exercise per day or we can live in a way that keeps natural movement relevant to us. The choice is ours.

Another thing to consider when discussing a proper movement routine is fascia. Fasciae are the connective tissues that hold us together. Unfortunately, fascia can get bound up in the body, especially if you move improperly or remain in static postures for long periods of time. As fascia binds up, people tend to experience pain as extra pressure is placed on joints, muscles are shortened, and joint motion decreased. An important part of any movement routine is restoring flexibility to your fasciae and muscles. To address many years of built-up muscle tension, a good deep tissue massage therapist or myofascial therapist can come in handy. However, I believe it is even more important to focus on functional movement exercise that will increase flexibility and take your joints through their full range of motion. Things like yoga and foam rolling routines are useful tools to keeping your body loose and able to move through full range of motion.

Sometimes, even if we do focus on functional movements or restoring fascia, life just has other plans, and we get built-up pressure in our muscles and joints. At this point, as a chiropractor, I think that chiropractic adjustments can be very useful. Chiropractors specialize in creating joint space or joint motion where it has been decreased. Many times muscles get tight because our joints have lost motion or we have lost the correct curves in our spine which create an imbalance of pressure on the structures of the body. Since our muscles are also protectors, they get into a chronic state of protection when this happens; we tend to call this tightness or stiffness. Creating motion in those joints can not only free up trapped structures, triggering the muscles to relax and reducing inflammation and pain,[28] but they can also restore communication from our brain to our organs by freeing up trapped nerves.[29] Adjustments that increase joint motion can help us in our quest to achieve healthy overall movement, especially if we have gone long periods of time in our lives with little or no movement practices.

When most people think about movement they think about big movements of our arms and legs or types of movement seen in various types of exercise. As a chiropractor I spend a lot of time thinking about and treating movement at a segmental (joint by joint) level. There are many examples of how we have put our bodies in an environment that affects individual joint movement but none more visible than in the foot. Our feet have evolved to have a perfect interaction with the earth. The three arches of the foot provide us with the structural support we need. That is, unless we intervene by putting our feet in restrictive footwear that modify and weaken the foot.[30]

If you look at the foot of a baby, it is shaped like a wedge, wider at the toes and narrow at the heel. If you look at most adult feet they look very different. A lifetime of wearing shoes has narrowed and lifted the toes, weakened the arches (because they cannot fully splay out when the foot contacts the ground), and tightened the calf because many shoes have a raised heel. The combination of these things has led to the many lower body musculoskeletal aches and pains that plague our society.

Supporting the arches of our feet in the proper way will give us movement in our feet much closer to that of our ancestors, and insoles with "arch support" are not how we do this. If you look at arches that have been built, from ancient civilizations to modern bridges, they are supported at the ends where gravity pushes all the way through them. The design of the arch combined with the forces of the earth give us a solid structure. By wearing shoes we alter this dynamic, mainly by messing with the ends of the arches in our feet, which are now a raised heel and toes that angle in toward the midline. This alters the pressure we get from the ends of our feet and results in collapsed arches. A common "solution" to this is to wear arch support insoles, but they support the arches in your feet in the middle, which is not where the force support of an arch should come from. I once had a foot scan done and they told me that the lateral arches in my feet were weak (what years of soccer cleats will do to you) and they recommended custom orthotics. I couldn't help but wonder why they were telling me that to solve my foot problem I should put something in my shoes that would keep my foot in the exact same flawed state.

Obviously, modern society has made it very hard to go around without shoes, and the endless concrete we have created is hard on the joints. But this does not mean that we need to wear shoes that restrict the normal motion of our feet and shape them in unnatural ways. Rather, it means that we need to have footwear with padding that still allows our feet to do what they are supposed to do while protecting us from all those hard manmade surfaces. There are great companies like Vivobarefoot and Lems that are making this kind of footwear. Long story short, modern shoes are just one way we have restricted the normal motion of individual joints in our body, and in this case it ends up altering the normal motion of our body as a whole. For more information about feet and proper foot motion check out Dr. Ray McLanahan, a.k.a. The Barefoot Podiatrist.

The last thing to note before I give you my recommendations for movement frequency is that it is much easier to achieve that healthy fit body we desire when we are eating a nutrient rich diet. I know, I know—again with the diet. But it truly is the single most important thing. If you get your diet pretty spot on you will find that you don't have to work as hard as everyone thinks to stay fit. After years of doing core exercises—some of them healthy, like planks, and others not so healthy, like crunches—it was only when I started eating a diet similar to our ancient ancestors that my abdominal muscles showed up. It's too bad, because I would have welcomed their lady-impressing powers many times before then!

So what do I recommend for movement? Well I think that 1-2 sessions of burst movement exercises per week is a good idea. These burst movements could be interval sets of functional resistance exercises and perhaps some sprints or intervals of cardio, but burst movement should only be done for 20-30 minutes in a session. Then, I suggest 2-3 sessions of lengthening or flexibility exercises per week. This could be yoga and foam rolling. The most important aspect of a movement routine is to stay moving. In general, in times while you are not formally working out, you should be moving your body. If you have to work at a desk then get a standing desk, sit on an exercise ball to force yourself to engage your core while working, or find a way to do your work while sitting on the floor to put your hips through greater range of motion. Get up and walk the halls every half hour. Just stay moving. Continuing to do the same behaviors (like excessive sitting or looking down at our phones) that cause imbalances and restricted movement and then attempting to use functional movement to combat the bad behavior is like fighting fires set by an arsonist without trying to catch the arsonist.

So how is movement going to help us save our species and our planet? Natural movements will help us build stronger genes so that the next generation is stronger and better adapted to survive. If we truly look for ways to stay moving in our daily life we may find that it is practical to ride our bike to work, or maybe even walk. That sounds like something people do for the environment, but remember that is just a side effect. We are selfishly doing it for our own health. Maybe we could at least walk to the bus stop and then walk to work when we get off the bus. Finding ways to incorporate movement into our life can help us reduce the amount of toxicity we put into our air. Finally, exercise is the single best treatment for depression, and so incorporating movement into our lives will create a better personal environment for us all by creating happier people.

To recap some of the recommendations of this section, begin to focus on the kind of functional, full range of motion body movement our ancestors would have naturally experienced every day. Look into burst training. Consider massage or chiropractic adjustment for restoring motion you may already have lost. And, if you can, choose footwear that will allow your feet their full range of movement. For more about improving your movement I suggest checking out the book, *Move Your DNA,* by Katy Bowman and *The Functional Movement Handbook* by Craig Leibenson.

Stress

A few years ago I had a very pleasant and fun to talk with 64-year-old patient. We will call her Mary. Mary's main complaint was that two to three times a week she was experiencing headaches that she described as "shocks." These shocks would make her unable to do much of anything; she would have to go into a dark room and wait until they subsided. I treated her like I would anyone else who was suffering from what seemed to be migraines. We did some gut healing and gave her various high quality supplements like magnesium. She was an experienced gardener so she was getting plenty of good food, but we did start to incorporate more high quality fats into her diet, and I started adjusting her full spine. To help her detoxify and build healthy mitochondria, she even bought a far-infrared sauna, which her and her husband both starting using.

Despite some decreased intensity of the shocks, at our four-month visit she came in saying she had been getting worse. As we started talking about what was going on and some strategies to approach it, she eventually gave me some information that she had neglected to tell me at our first visit, despite the fact that I had asked about stressful events in her life. She told me that she had a daughter who had gotten married about eight years ago and moved to the other side of the country. Unfortunately, her daughter's marriage had turned into a physically abusive one. After some time, Mary was unable to contact her daughter for several weeks and so she filed a missing person's report. Her daughter, it turns out, had been in hiding from her husband and, regrettably, when the police found her, the first person they contacted was her husband. By the time Mary walked into my office, three years had already passed with no further contact from her daughter, and for two of those she had been experiencing the shocks. The stress of her situation was most likely the main contributor to the shocks. Psychological stress can be a major proponent in any chronic condition or ailment.

Although most of us don't go through this type of stress every day, we are all familiar with stress and feel it on a daily basis; it is inevitable in today's world. Stress is a normal reaction to our environment, however, it has almost become the default way of life for many people—so much so that when we don't feel stressed; we may feel that we are not being productive enough. Countless times I have asked someone how their day or week has been and they sigh and say, "Busy, but busy is good." I often think to myself that judging just by the tone of their response, it doesn't sound too good. We seem to think that all stress is inevitable, and we should just accept it and persevere; yet we also hear all the time that managing our stress is good for us. So which is it? In reality, it's a little of both. Some stress *is* unavoidable, and we should learn how to manage it, but not all of it is necessary. I feel that managing stress is the most often ignored component of healthy living. Because of the nature of how stress affects us, it is hard to see its direct repercussions and even harder to link certain disease processes to it. Let's take a closer look at stress.

There is mostly a negative connotation to stress, but it can be good in some ways. Stress is just a stimulus that causes us to react to our environment; it is one aspect of what drives evolution, and without it evolution would not be able to push forward. Stress has always been there for every species, and since it is necessary for evolution, we will probably never live stress-free lives. I've heard the argument that our stress today must be way less than our ancestors experienced living out in the natural world. This was concluded on the premise that today we are not constantly worrying about finding food or whether or not there is a lion around the next corner. Because humans have largely evolved in the world that existed up until 10,000 years ago, our stress response is set up for life in the wild, and, as discussed in Chapter 8, that response gets little relief in today's world.

In studying animals on the African savannah, Stanford biologist Robert Sapolsky found that the animals' stress cycles were a little different from the stress cycles of humans living in the modern world. He showed this by measuring cortisol, which is the hormone many living beings release in response to stressful situations. In zebras he found that cortisol levels are normal while they are grazing and just minding their own business. This changes rapidly when a predator comes out of the brush—their cortisol spikes in response to this stimulus, and it stays elevated throughout the chase. If they escape, he found that as soon as the zebras are safe, their cortisol returns to normal almost immediately. This shows that zebras, and many other animals in the wild, are only having stress responses when absolutely necessary. This is probably why the book is called *Why Zebras Don't Get Ulcers* and *why* dancing zebras adorn the front cover.

Well, so what? Why does this study matter? It matters because if you study a modern world human, especially those in the West, we see something somewhat different. Our stress response is pretty much the same as what we see in wild mammals, which makes sense because we evolved in the wild just like they did. The difference is that our response doesn't always turn off as it does for zebras. We may not have to worry about getting away from predators too often, but we do have constant stressors in our lives every day. Things like keeping your job, passing that test, moving up in your company, sitting in traffic, and making sure your family has everything it needs are never ceasing sources of stress. These constant stressors result in chronic elevated levels of the stress hormone cortisol. It is important to note that this is different than what you feel when a co-worker jumps out from behind the water cooler to scare you—the response you feel from that is high levels of adrenaline (signaled to be secreted by cortisol) rushing through your system. The chronic stress we experience every day is what people feel when they say they are having a stressful day, and they have chronic levels of elevated stress hormones. This becomes a problem when that stressful day goes on day after day after day.

Our stress response system should go back to its non-stress levels after a stressful experience. However, we tend to perceive never-ending stressors in our world and our bodies tends to stay In a chronic low level elevation of cortisol, which is not something they are evolved to deal with. It has been shown that prolonged elevated cortisol levels are indicators of digestive problems, high blood pressure, insulin resistance, sexual dysfunction, and chronic inflammation.[31] When our body secretes cortisol, the brain prepares us to fight or flee and other bodily processes are shut down temporarily. The symptoms of chronic elevated cortisol make sense, because when in the state of "flee the scene as fast as possible," the body is not concerned about digestion, metabolism, reproducing, or rest. High blood pressure and inflammation also make sense, because the body is using those mechanisms to force blood to areas that can help us fight or flee.

Aside from shutting down basic human functions, this chronic elevated stress response creates an imbalance in the nervous system. The nervous system has two different extremes that we are constantly balancing between. Those extremes are the parasympathetic and sympathetic nervous systems, and we are always somewhere in between one extreme or the other. Your parasympathetic nervous system is your "rest and digest" system, and we should be in this state most of the time, just like the zebra grazing on the savannah. Your sympathetic nervous system is the "fight or flight" system, and we should move more in its direction when we are sensing danger. Many people in our society are stuck continually in fight or flight because of the constant bombardment of stresses, creating decreased tone in their parasympathetic systems. This means that we are weakening our ability to get back into a rest and digest state.

This can be illustrated by comparing it to driving a manual gear-shifting car. Let's pretend that you have a manual car that represents your rest and digest nervous system. If we drive that car for a year we would get very used to the clutch on that car. Then let's say that we go through a year of stress; this year will be represented by being forced to drive a different manual car, which represents our fight or flight nervous system. Anyone who has driven different manual cars knows that the clutch feels different at first. Having this stress at first is very apparent. As we continue through our year of stress, that new clutch starts to feel normal to us—stress becomes normal. A year later, let's say that we finally can go back to driving the *rest and digest* car. Unfortunately, when we try and go back to using the clutch in that car, it doesn't feel normal; the stress car feels more normal, even though it is not. You have been in a stress state so long that you have a decreased ability to drive the *rest and digest* car. Staying in the stress response nervous system so long that it decreases our ability to find the so-called relax nervous system contributes to many of the health issues we see today.

One of the best ways to increase your body's ability to go back into parasympathetic mode is to stimulate the vagus nerve. This nerve originates in your brain and goes to all the internal organs, including the heart. One of the most surprising results of decreased tone of the parasympathetic system is a heart attack. A little known fact is that when autopsies are done on heart attack victims, the majority of them do not have a blockage or clot anywhere in the arteries supplying the heart. This is because blood clots are actually an uncommon cause of heart attacks. The more common cause is the decrease in tone of the parasympathetic nervous system which, when it hits a certain point, sends us into a cascade of reactions that cause the symptoms we know as a heart attack.[32] You may be wondering about cholesterol at this point. Well, cholesterol has never been the cause of heart disease; it's actually very good for you, and clots of cholesterol just don't happen frequently enough to explain the high amount of heart attacks we see. The chronic stimulation of sympathetic activity and the suppression of parasympathetic activity is the root cause behind most heart attacks.[33] So this means that heart attacks, the second leading cause of death in America (after our medical system), are not the root cause of death—stress is. For more mind-blowing information about the heart, check out *Human Heart, Cosmic Heart* by Dr. Thomas Cowan.

So, what are we going to do about all this stress? Hacking stress is one of the hardest tasks I have with my patients because I feel that the many stress management techniques, while useful, are not actually fixing the problem. When I try to fix stress issues I try to attack them at the source and then equip the patient with stress management techniques to use in times that just get a little too crazy. To me the answer to our stress problem is three-fold.

The first tool to address is diet—bet you didn't see that one coming. A nutrient-rich diet will provide your body with the materials it needs to better cope with the daily bombardment of stress. There are many foods that are termed adaptogenic in the health world, and these are foods, or herbs, that help us have a healthy response to stress. In other words they help us respond to stress more like those wild zebras. Some foods and herbs can be seen as medicinal, such as turmeric, which is known to reduce inflammation, or ginger, to help fight off a cold. But mostly I don't like describing food as medicine. Anything we can ingest is just providing us nutrients; some foods have more of certain nutrients that help our bodies perform certain tasks. The only reason we see certain foods as medicinal is that we have gone so far away from eating real food that when we start eating it and our body heals we say that this food must have medicinal properties. Health is not created by any type of medicine, whether it's pharmaceutical or food; health is the default state of our body when it has the tools it needs to function inside and out.

The second approach to stress is to start taking steps to simplify your life. This may sound unrealistic because of everything that our world says that we "need" to have or do to be functional in society, but I have found that if we really think about it, there are lots of things in our lives that we could live without. That goes for possessions, lifestyles, and responsibilities. I feel that I live a pretty simple life, but I didn't do that on purpose. Growing up, my family wasn't poor but we were far from rich. When I turned eighteen I became a student and remained one until I was twenty-eight. Students don't have much cash, and in those ten years I learned to live with only what I needed. Even when I traveled to Central America I took not even one backpack full of stuff despite bumming around for three and a half months. My point is that my minimalist life just happened. I got very used to not having many things, having as uncomplicated a lifestyle as I could, and still doing the things that were expected of me without taking on too much. Every time I moved I would go through my things, and if I hadn't used it while I lived at that house, I wouldn't take it to the new one—with very little exceptions. We don't need a ton of possessions, complicated lifestyles, and excess responsibilities to give us what we need to survive. For more information on this approach I suggest looking into Joshua Fields Millburn and Ryan Nicodemus, who call themselves The Minimalists and are owning this particular approach to stress reduction.

The third strategy is to change our perception about what constitutes a stressful situation. The zebras only had stress responses when they were experiencing life threatening situations. I bet if we take a step back and think about our daily stressors, some of them are just not as "life-ending" as they seem. I feel that the state of society is such that we are terrified of possible futures because we are told to be terrified, or our peers are scared of certain things happening, and so we become scared, too. However, most of us perhaps haven't asked ourselves, *what happens if we chose not to be terrified anymore?* What happens if we attempt to regain control of our own lives rather than be controlled by fear? I am reminded of a story I once read—the story of the five monkeys.

> Once upon a time there was some very cruel research done to five monkeys in a cage. They were locked in and

given very poor quality food and water. In the middle of the cage there was a ladder and at the top of that ladder a bunch of exquisite bananas, but whenever one monkey would try to climb the ladder to reach the bananas all the monkeys would get sprayed with high-pressured freezing water. After this happened many times, they learned the bananas were off limits. Because all of them got sprayed if one tried to get the bananas, the monkeys started holding each other accountable, always stopping that one determined son of a gun from trying to climb the ladder. Animal cruelty didn't stop there. They now took one monkey out of the cage and replaced him with another monkey, who had no idea what had been going on. Once he got in there he looked around and was like, *seriously guys, don't you know there are bananas up there*, and he went for them. When he started to climb the ladder all the other monkeys got angry, start yelling and attacking him in order to prevent everyone from getting punished with the freezing water. Eventually, the new guy learned that those bananas were off limits. The researchers kept replacing monkeys until none of the original monkeys were left in the cage. Each time the same thing happened. Eventually, none of the monkeys in the cage had experienced the negative consequences, yet still lived in fear because of how they were told their world works. Unfortunately, I see very similar things going on in human society today.

The moral of the story is that we should start taking control of our stress/fear responses instead of letting them control us. Behaving with fear or stress just because everyone else is behaving that way is counterproductive to achieving a life that creates health.

One strategy to changing our perception of stress is to shift how we react to things that may happen around us. For instance, let's say you are driving down the road and someone swerves through traffic and cuts you off without using their blinker. Since this is one of your pet peeves you are irate with this person, and it sends you into an anger spiral for most of the day. It could be helpful to realize that, in this situation, the person who cut you off does not have the problem, you have the problem. The person in the car is just fine, probably going about their day with no anger spiral. Should he have done what he did? No, probably not, but reacting with anger the way many people do does not change something that is out of our control. By reacting in anger we are showing that the problem with the situation is our own. The point is that we should not be consumed by a stressful response to things that are out of our control, and we should do this for the sake of our own health. I realized this early on in my clinical career when I would see patients who I deemed as unhealthy. I thought that they had a problem in that they were unhealthy, but most of them didn't have a problem with how they were; I was the one who had the problem. The problem only became theirs when they wanted to start to make changes in their health. I learned that I should educate them as much as I could but recognize that the decision to achieve better health was theirs and not mine.

Another contributor to how we perceive stress these days—one that we can decrease our exposure to—is the media. Whether or not you believe that what the media reports is accurate is not what I'm concerned about here. I'm talking about the fact that we even have media in the first place. This has been a dramatic change for humans in very recent history. Nowadays, if something bad happens in a very distant part of the world, we see it on the news within hours, and we become stressed out about it. If the news wasn't there it would have had no effect on us, and we would just have gone on with our day with no issues. I understand that having access to news and fast transmission of information across the world can be very useful in some ways, but having access to and having to handle such a vast amount of information every day contributes to our heightened levels of cortisol. Our ability to adapt to stress did not evolve to handle the stress of an entire planet.

My point here is that maybe we can alter how we get our information to have a better personal and community health outcomes. Everyone has a right to, and should be, informed, but maybe we should stick to the local news and newspapers rather than having negative emotional reactions to things that happen so far away from us that it becomes counterproductive for us to even know about them. Aside from unfortunate things like natural disasters, where we all should help those affected, no matter how far away, it might be useful for us do some media dieting. Maybe even restrict our news to once a day rather than having it stress us out as soon as it pops up on our phone. Also, it can be useful to do some research about things we hear on the news before we react to them. Getting the whole picture is very important. Implementing these strategies will not only help create a health-promoting environment for the individual but create a less stressed out society as a whole.

Even with those three approaches to navigating our stressful world there are still unavoidable sources of stress, and so we need to understand what to do to reduce our elevated cortisol and return to a *rest and digest* state. The most appropriate way to do this, as far as living in a way closest to our ancient ancestors, is to get out in nature and soak it up. Research has shown being in green spaces, or other natural environments, has a dramatic effect on your cortisol levels.[34] Amazingly, it showed that those who spent a day in nature had lower cortisol levels on average, and not just for the day but for weeks following their nature excursion. It turns out that everything we hear, see, smell, and touch out in nature has a calming effect on our bodies while the things we sense in an urban landscape send alert signals throughout our bodies. Just think of the effects that would result from being in an urban environment all the time. This is proof that the natural world is the world we are most adapted to be in. It is important to point out, however, that we should not see nature as a therapy. The symptoms we see from stress are a result of us having been removed from our natural environment, which is nature. How could what is natural for us be a therapy?

The lowering of cortisol by spending time in nature is just one way we can increase our parasympathetic tone, which, as we discussed earlier, is a major player in preventing heart attacks. Dr. Thomas Cowan sums up how to create a healthy parasympathetic nervous system:

> Nourishing our parasympathetic nervous system means dismantling a way of life for which humans are ill suited. This way of life, in my view, is industrial civilization. The known things that nourish our parasympathetic nervous system are contact with nature, loving relations, trust, economic security, and sex—in a sense, a whole new world.

Aside from those tools, there are also many other forms of stress management that you can use to combat inevitable stress without too much effort. You can try everything from learning to meditate, to engaging in a stress-reducing hobby, to participating in different forms of spirituality. There are a number of meditation practices you can learn; you can even download a meditation app on your phone. You can try neurofeedback or find a heart math practitioner. These are particularly useful tools because you will get feedback that can help you deal with stress in the future rather than just conquering your current bout of stress and then having to deal with another episode the very next day.

All of these approaches can help you get back into that parasympathetic state so you can stop being jealous of zebras and be more like our ancient ancestors. So how does this help us save our species? Well, as I have said, we evolved over millions of years fairly selfishly; we had to think of the survival of our genes to the exclusion of everyone else's. However, humans have also developed a sense of community, and while I think it is important for health to try and create an environment that is more like our ancient ancestors, I think that this is one case where we should take advantage of the bit of unselfishness and cooperation we have developed.

Therefore, if we all got a handle on our stress and stopped responding to all the stressful, dividing stimuli seen in the media and throughout our communities, I feel that we would be less hostile to the world around us. We would be much more likely to help and cooperate with others. Right now many of us are caught up in stress responses to what we are told we need to fear, and we let it consume and change us. I feel that a society with control over stress and absence of unnecessary fear would be one that could come together and solve the biggest problems facing us as a species.

Spirituality

I find it hard to believe that our ancient wild ancestors were very spiritual. There is some archeological evidence that late in the human evolutionary game, right before we adapted agriculture, some groups of our human predecessors practiced rituals and burial of their dead. For the most part, however, I think that the millions of years of evolution happened without much spirituality. We were just another animal in the wild and although some animals in nature show us that they have emotions, as far as I know they do not gather together to perform any type of ritual or spiritual practice—unless you are watching the opening scene of *The Lion King*. In that case, cue the epic Lion King music and let's get this ritual started.

In my humble opinion—and this is only an opinion—spirituality and religion only started gaining force once we came together in larger groups about 10,000 years ago. The reason for this is because humans started working together to achieve "better" living conditions and "easier" lives. In order for us to be successful in this all the members had to be working together toward a common goal. Looking back, it is amazing we were able to do this at all, given that we had just spent millions of years evolving to selfishly live for the success of only our genes. As we moved toward a life of agriculture, evolution slowly started to favor groups of humans with the behavior genes that made them more cooperative in large groups. Those evolutionarily selected groups of humans started to adopt common beliefs that offered explanations and ethical guidelines for the way we lived and acted. These common beliefs made it possible for large groups of humans to unite for the purpose of achieving the common goal of survival.

As we have discussed, once agriculture was adopted, human populations grew, and evolution would have created whole populations with genes for strong cooperation and the ability to unite under common belief. Eventually those groups became large enough that they overcrowded and outnumbered those still living out in the wild—the cooperative genes were triumphant. This doesn't mean that our selfishness would have been completely eliminated; it's just that those who were a little less selfish were more likely to survive because they could combine forces with others. This whole process would have resulted in the eventual development of common beliefs systems like religions. Therefore, religions evolved just like any other human trait or characteristic. Using this thinking it is ironic that those most opposed to evolution because of their religious beliefs in fact only have religious beliefs because of evolution.

To conclude, I do not think religion is necessary when trying to restore health by creating an environment similar to ancient humans. Yes, spirituality has become a big part of what differentiates humans from all other species. However, it is ironic (and frankly sad) that religion—one of the things that originally brought us closer together to cooperate in large groups—is now one of the most dividing aspects of our society. Differences in religion or spirituality have been the result of so much violence and death within the short history of humans. Why this violence happens is confusing to me because there are thousands of religions in the world today and thousands more that have gone extinct throughout human history and not a single one is "right." It's pointless to keep fighting about whose god is the true god. In my opinion organized religion has created as many problems as the concept of race, which is another human invented concept, and one used to exploit others for individual gain. Growing up, I remember thinking that Jewish and Muslim were races of people. When I discovered that they weren't, and that I could become Jewish or Muslim if I wanted, I was shocked. Often, we don't even understand the interwoven histories of the labels we are using, and that goes for both religion and race. Humans tend toward a binary system—us versus them—within which we determine that something or someone is one way or another, with no possible in between. That kind of binary thinking may have helped us succeed in the wild—when individual competition largely determined who survived and who did not—but within the context of a society of human beings, it is tearing us apart.

I am not opposed to religion or religious people. The way I look at differences in religion or spirituality is that if whatever you believe helps and motivates you to do good things in this world, or helps you have a healthy optimistic outlook of the world, then by all means go with it. However, if you find that believing what you do causes you to judge others who believe in something different, or be skeptical of someone based on their beliefs, or make you feel like you're better than other people who think differently than you, then take a step back and ask yourself some tough questions: is your belief just selfishly motivated thinking? Is it making your world, and the world of those around you, a better place, or is it driving you apart from your fellow humans? I would ask you to realize that just because you have found what works for you, do not assume that everyone needs to have that in their life as well. There is more than one way to be a good person and find peace in this world. Spirituality is an individual journey. If you like to take your individual journey and share it with others on Sunday mornings, great. If you like to meditate on your own or be in touch with the power of the natural world, that is also great. In the end, we should choose who we associate with by comparing how similarly we interact with the world, not by having the same belief structure and/or label.

Despite all the issues that organized religion creates for the masses, from a health perspective various means of spirituality do offer many individuals stress reduction techniques and motivation to do good things in our society. Spirituality is an amazing way of coping with the unnatural stresses of our modern day life.

If we start to look at our various approaches to spirituality as different approaches to the same goal—to create a better world—I feel that the divisiveness we experience from organized forms of spirituality today will drop significantly. We will all be less closed off to those who don't label themselves the same way, and therefore, be more willing to learn from various spiritual paths in order to come together and tackle the big problems that our species is facing.

Light

I am not an expert in the physics of light, nor do I know all the ins and outs of how all the different types of light affect us, but I do know that for millions of years humans watched the sun rise and fall, day after day. As you could probably guess, our physiology became pretty responsive to that consistent stimulus and that consistent type of light. You can see this by testing your cortisol levels throughout the day. Aside from being the hormone that helps us respond to stress it also regulates our sleep wake cycle, our circadian rhythm. In response to light exposure at sunrise, our cortisol spikes in the morning and dips down in the evening when the sun goes to bed. These days, due to the invention of artificial light, this balance is disrupted constantly. *Thanks,* Edison. Even when we discovered fire it started to affect our circadian rhythm. However, fire is much more natural and doesn't cause near the harm that artificial light does, plus the benefit of being able to cook our food and provide us warmth far outweighed the minimal cost.

The problem with man-made light is that it does not expose us to the full spectrum of light, and this limited spectrum of light has detrimental effects on our body. But Edison's revolutionary invention of the original light bulb wasn't so bad compared to what was to come. Once single spectrum blue lights came about in the form of LEDs, compact fluorescents, and anything with a screen—computer, TV, cell phone—our environments became extremely polluted with unnatural light. One of the effects of blue light is that it can suppress melatonin, the sleep hormone.[35] So if you spend the last few hours before bed looking at a screen and then have trouble getting to sleep, it's time to change your before bedtime activity. Sleep is much more important than we realize.

In his book, *Why We Sleep,* Matthew Walker gives many examples of the effect getting quality sleep can have. In Edina, Minnesota the school start time was shifted from 7:35 AM to 8:30 AM, allowing students to get more sleep and to get sleep that is more in line with their biological rhythms. The result was that the average verbal SAT scores went from 605 the year before the change to 761 after the change. Average math SAT scores went from 683 to 739. In another school district in Minnesota they shifted their start time from 7:30 AM to 8:00 AM and saw a 60% reduction in traffic accidents among 16 to 18-year-old drivers in their county. If getting a little more sleep can have this much impact, imagine what getting better quality sleep by decreasing blue light could do.

You can imagine that if artificial light is bad for us then natural light must be better. In fact, natural sunlight is essential for life. Plants can't live without it and neither can animals. Sunlight in the right quantities is very healthy for humans; we use natural light exposure to regulate a natural sleep-wake cycle, make Vitamin D, boost fertility, and regenerate our energy-making structures (mitochondria). Exposure to as much natural light as you can get without getting burned is a must for health. Obviously, when you get sunburn, especially repeated sunburn, it increases risk of things like skin cancer. However, using sunscreen that is full of toxicants raises your risk of skin cancer just as much or more. Not only are our sunscreens polluting our bodies, they are heavily polluting our oceans as they seep into the water we are swimming in. One of the best ways to protect yourself from the sun is to boost your body's natural sun protection by eating a nutrient-rich diet (I had to sneak diet in one last time!) while also using safer alternatives to sunscreen like lighter, body covering clothing. If you must use some sort of sunscreen, then you can check out the Environmental Working Group website to see which sunscreens are the least toxic or find natural or mineral based sunscreens that will not expose your skin to as many harsh chemicals.

The obvious way to get back into a light environment that is more like our natural environment would be to minimize your exposure to excess artificial light, especially after the sun goes down, and by replacing artificial light with safe amounts of natural sunlight—focus especially on replacing blue light. Switch your CFLs (the curly bulbs) back to the old clear incandescent bulbs. Avoid staring at screens as much as possible. You can even get covers for your screens that help block blue light, and I suggest avoiding screens altogether two hours before bed. This will help protect your eyes from damage, help you get better sleep, and help get you back on a normal sleep-wake cycle so you don't wake up feeling so groggy. You could even get a fireplace or candles for the evenings because fire is so nice and cozy. Be safe though. Smokey the Bear says only you can prevent house fires...and insomnia.

For more on the effects that light has on our health please visit www.mercola.com and educate yourself with the numerous articles and interviews Dr. Mercola has on light.

Electromagnetic Fields

We are all electrical beings. We are full of positive and negative ions that create electrical charges in and around each and every cell. When our brain wants to send a message anywhere in the body, it is sent via an electrical signal that travels through our nerves. Because we are electromagnetic beings we each have our own electromagnetic field surrounding us. In nature the only places we would have encountered other electromagnetic fields would be with other living things and the natural electromagnetic field of the earth. If you pay attention you will find that your body can pick up on other living things that come close to you without using your sense of touch, taste, hearing, smell, or vision. Most of us can remember a time when we could sense that someone was near us before we could see or hear them. The most common for me is when someone tries to hide somewhere and scare me as a prank. Whenever someone has done this to me, the second right before they reveal themselves I have this feeling that something in my environment is off.

I remember when I was living in Ireland and I would ride my bike to work every day, there was a section of my route where I had to ride on a single lane path that crossed over the intersection of two highways. This path was deserted most days, but occasionally there was someone walking on the path, going the same direction in which I was going. Since it was very loud, due to all the traffic driving on the highway, if there was someone walking on the path they could not hear me coming up behind them on my bike. Interestingly, I'd say 9 times out of 10, when I got up behind them they would turn their head, see me there, and politely move aside so I could go past them. For months I tried to figure out how most of them could tell I was there. Did Irish people have super-powered ears? Were they being warned by magical leprechauns? I settled on the fact that they could feel my electromagnetic field come into their own, much like when you are in a quiet bookstore and you sense that someone has come up behind you, and the hairs stand up on the back of your neck.

Obviously, I don't know if this is actually what was happening to me in Ireland, but we do know that we each emit an electromagnetic field, and research has shown that our electro-magnetic bodies are affected by the growing numbers of electromagnetic fields in our tech savvy environment.[37] Any electrical device will give off an electromagnetic field that has a negative impact on our own, but those with a wireless signal are much more detrimental. Obviously, if we lived in our natural environment we would only have the electromagnetic contact of other life forms and the earth. Since we live in a very different world than that of an ancient human, we come into contact with all kinds of technologies that also have electromagnetic fields, such as big machinery, electric or hybrid cars, computers, cell phones, cell phone towers, wi-fi, and anything wireless.

Researchers in Germany, Israel, and Austria have found profound detrimental effects to people living close to cell phone towers. The German study concluded that, "the risk of newly developing cancer was three times higher among those patients who had lived during the past ten years within a distance of 400m from the cellular transmitter in comparison to those who had lived further away." The Israeli study showed "significantly greater incidence of cancers" and the Austrian study showed "significant cancer incidence" among those living in the vicinity of cell phone towers.[38,39,40]

These studies are alarming, and while they give us some insight into the danger, we don't even know the full effect that these electromagnetic fields will have on humans who have been exposed to them for their entire lives. I fear that the repercussions will be dramatic. It used to be that we knew that these signals had an effect, but we didn't know why. It was thought that damage was caused because of a heating up of the tissues. That was until Dr. Martin Pall looked a little deeper. He found it interesting that the group of heart medications known as calcium channel blockers seemed to mitigate the damage of EMFs (one positive among the array of negatives this drug can do). Following this clue he eventually found that EMFs caused damage by opening voltage gated calcium channels, allowing calcium to flood into the cells. He found that this phenomenon caused "a whole series of biological changes," including "oxidative stress; single and double stranded breaks in cellular DNA; therapeutic effects; blood-brain barrier breakdown; greatly depressed melatonin levels and sleep disruption; cancer; male and female infertility; immune dysfunction; neurological dysfunction; cardiac dysfunction including tachycardia, arrhythmia and sudden cardiac death."[41] Dr. Pall says that, "A two-phase program for greatly improving EMF safety standards is proposed."

Those kinds of effects are pretty scary, especially when we don't even know what the effects of lifetime exposure to these signals will be. Just like light, though, there are bad types of EMF and good types. The EMFs from other living things and from Earth are actually healing and are the reason why contact with nature and human touch are so healing. There is even technology out there called Pulsed Electromagnetic Frequency (PEMF) that can be used as therapy to expose our body to the right type of EMFs. It has been shown to help with early wound healing[42] and increase bone growth in osteoporosis.[43]

As far as avoiding EMFs, it is really hard to completely get rid of the bad EMF signals that affect us everywhere we go while also functioning in a society that is so reliant on them. So hard in fact that it is nearly impossible for the average person to do. In order to bring our electromagnetic environment more in line with the natural environment we came from the best we can do is reduce the amount we are exposed to. Things we can do are turn off the wi-fi at our house at night, use speaker phone so as not to have the phone so close to our heads, connect with cords and wires whenever possible, and get shields that will protect us from the electromagnetic radiation coming from the devices we use. You can even hire a building biologist that will come to your home and find all the sources electromagnetic radiation in your home and suggest ways to decrease or eliminate them. This may seem tedious but remember, disease is death caused by a thousand cuts. The more cuts we can get rid of, the better chance we have to live a disease free life. None of us really knows the cut limit of our own bodies, so keeping the cut number low in any way that we can is important.

Genes

Lastly, I want to talk a little about genes. Hopefully, I have shown you that we have more control over our genes than Western medicine thinks we do. However, there are some things about genes that we cannot change and these can be useful to know when it comes to trying to achieve the greatest health possible. The information gathered from taking a look at our genes through genetic testing can be used to personalize each individual's strategy by incorporating aspects of their personal ancient ancestors' lives into their own. Obviously, no one's ancient ancestors would have had a way to examine their genes to find out if they had genetic weaknesses, but today we can combine this information with the wisdom of an ancient life to achieve health.

Genetic testing to look for variants in an individual's DNA that can affect the health advice they are given is growing in popularity. Be sure you seek out a knowledgeable practitioner for this. Some of the best I know of are practitioners who have been certified through the Apeiron Academy.

Practitioners

While many of these strategies can be done on your own, sometimes getting started can require a little help, especially for those people with complex chronic conditions. As we have discussed, looking for that help in the Western medicine system we have available to us is not the best option, and Western medicine should be relied on mainly in an emergency. So who do we go to instead? Well, I coach clients across the county through my online health coaching business at www.resourceyourhealth.com, and there are many knowledgeable practitioners who do the same. I use principles of functional medicine and my holistic study of the human body and mind to focus on identifying the most pertinent changes that need to be made, depending on the client's situation, so that they don't have to make all the changes listed above at once. I help people with all kinds of symptoms, but I specialize in helping people with heart disease, type 1 diabetes, digestive symptoms, and autoimmune disease. For all of my clients working to achieve health, changes are necessary—but I identify changes that are achievable and fit well within each individual's life as much as possible. I coach people into forming long-lasting habits that will create health for years to come, rather than one-off treatments that are short lived and keep clients relying on me.

Aside from that, there are many doctors who are starting to realize that the type of medicine they were taught in medical school is not effective for the disease epidemic we are seeing today. Many of those doctors have acquired extra knowledge and training to best treat their patients. Doing the things I suggested in this chapter are going to set you up for long term health, but the testing done by a knowledgeable functional medicine practitioner, while not always necessary, can be helpful in guiding your health journey. If you are someone who likes to be able to meet with a doctor in person then a doctor trained in functional medicine is a good place to start. Whether they realize it or not, functional medicine doctors are helping you reduce the amount of personal environmental change that we have been though as a species in the last 10,000 years. I myself studied functional medicine for a while before finally connecting the dots between that study and my interest in human history. After I made the connection, I could see clearly that functional medicine is so effective precisely because it makes our lives a little more like our ancient environment. My brain exploded with epiphany! A functional medicine doctor does not necessarily have to grasp this connection to be able to help you; functional medicine treatments are fundamentally based on moving us back to a more ancient lifestyle within the confines of our modern lives.

Doctors who are not trained in functional medicine can also sometimes be good options. There are naturopathic doctors and other health-conscious doctors that will take a "create health" approach as well, you just may have to spend a little time finding the right one. In general, a good strategy is to find a practitioner who sets a healthy example and is really passionate about achieving optimal health themselves as well as the optimal health of their patients. If your doctor is not passionate about what creates health for him or herself, then what makes you think they care about finding your optimal health? If your doctor's goal is not to make you less dependent on medication, or to get you off of it completely, then get out of there. Lastly, if you approach your doctor and tell them that you are going to start making changes to your lifestyle and they say that they don't want you off medications or are not interested in what you are doing, then you should fire your doctor and get a new one. You are paying them, and you deserve a treatment plan that will give you the best outcome. Don't be afraid to shop around for doctors to find one that will work with you and try and meet your needs as well as give you optimal health.

Finally, some brief thoughts on dentistry. The toxic way that dentistry has been practiced for too long is starting to be exposed. Many treatments that dentists perform cause more problems than they fix. These include amalgam fillings that leak neurotoxic mercury into our bodies, root canals which become a source of chronic infection, and improper removal of teeth which can also lead to chronic infections in the jawbone. The health of your mouth is so important to the overall health of your body. I am not a dentist, and I don't know everything about dental care; however, I can warn people about these harmful procedures as well as advocate for the amazing results I have seen from my patients going and getting their mouths cleaned up and toxin free. In general, if your dentist doesn't know who Dr. Weston Price or Dr. Hal Huggins are, and are not willing to look into their work for your sake, then you need to find a new dentist. You can go to www.hugginsappliedhealing.com to find one near you. You can also go to https://www.westonaprice.org/ for a great resource concerning dentistry and nutrition.

I realize that it is a hassle to change healthcare practitioners and to find ways to get quality care without it costing an arm and a leg. The way the system is set up forces many of those doctors who are passionate about their health and the health of their patients to run a practice that does not take insurance. It's a broken system. As much of a hassle as it may be, finding the right healthcare practitioners to guide you through the misinformed and ill-equipped world of healthcare can be a critical move when it comes to protecting the only life you have.

Concluding Thoughts

Before we move on, I want you to realize what you would actually be doing if you made the changes suggested above. I have tried to illustrate how divorcing ourselves from the natural world is having negative impacts on our health as well as the planet. But I want you to think about your body as its own little planet or ecosystem that you call home. It does us no good to go out of our way to try to protect planet Earth if we are sacrificing the individual "planet" that is each of us. If you are concerned about global warming, then do something about the global warming (excess inflammation) happening in your own body. If you are concerned about the amount of dirty energy (fossil fuels) we are burning and want to use more clean energy, then make sure your body is burning the cleanest energy (fat) that it can and work to heal your energy-making structures (mitochondria). If you are concerned about the massive loss of species happening in our world today, then concern yourself with the massive loss of species happening in your body (microbiome) right now. If you are concerned with the world becoming too toxic of a place to live, then concern yourself with avoiding and detoxing all the toxicants that are polluting your body. The same things that destroy our world are the things that destroy us. If we all took little steps and made changes one at a time to control our health, then we would be taking huge steps to saving our home, because if we all created the best environment for bodies, it would make Earth a better environment for all living things.

We have gone through some of the most important areas for shifting back toward a more natural lifestyle, and how that can impact our personal and global environment. Now, it is important to note that we have been removed from our natural environment for a long time. Therefore, when you start to take steps back toward our natural environment it is going to take a little bit of rehabilitation time. For example, if you switched to footwear that encouraged more natural foot mechanics, some rehabilitation aches and pains in your feet should be expected. When I was in Costa Rica I spent some time at the Jaguar Rescue Center where the goal was to rehabilitate animals that had been raised in captivity back into their natural environment. The Center would take the howler monkeys in rehabilitation on daily trips out into the jungle so they could interact with the wild troops of monkeys that were passing by. Eventually, individual monkeys would learn how to live among wild peers and be accepted by a troop, thereby becoming rehabilitated. Among the staff at the rehabilitation center, it was basic knowledge that this process would take a long time. So when trying to get closer to a human's natural environment, be patient with your body as it rehabilitates to the changes you make.

As an example, let's say you wanted to start wearing less restrictive shoes or start going barefoot more often. That's great, just know that your feet have been cooped up in shoes since you were able to walk and the muscles in your feet are probably weak, or at least not used to being used in this different way. We seem to have it in our heads that if our feet hurt it is because they are not "supported" enough, when in reality shoes have been keeping feet from doing what they are evolved to do. Your hands and feet are how we most commonly interact with our environment and closing our feet off from the world is like trying to have a productive day with mittens on our hands. If we wore mittens on our hands every day for a long time we would lose function in our hands, just like we have lost strength in our feet. Therefore, it is going to take some time for you to gain the strength and dexterity to be able to go barefoot as well as adjust to a different diet, detoxify from stored toxins, and learn how to address your stress. Be patient and know that making these transitions is not always the most fun. Just remember the end product is well worth it.

If you do all the things I have discussed in this chapter you are setting yourself up for vibrant health. Thinking about making all those changes at once can be overwhelming, and I don't advocate that drastic of an approach. Looking at your life and changing things that you can, and when you can, will start you on the path to health; just continue to make changes that move you in a positive direction on that path. When you get stuck or loose motivation, find others doing the same thing you are—your tribe—and reach out to them. We are stronger together.

Chapter 17: Healing Myself

When it comes to trying a new approach to healing, my first patient has always been myself. I have come a long way since first becoming interested in health back when I was 20 years old, but I am not done, and I will always be taking strides to better my health. Most of the chronic diseases I have suffered from in my life are gone now; even my severe cat allergies seem to have disappeared, as our cats Jeff, Louis, and Alfred can cuddle against my face without provoking the itchy eyes, runny nose, and sneezing I had come to expect. It was not an easy path to healing my ailments, and it took years of trial and error to figure out why my body was so ill and what to do in order to allow it to heal.

Through those years I tried many things, many of them totally wrong, and my progression to the way I live my life now was slow. I started out thinking that just eating more fruits and vegetables was how you stayed healthy and that bad things in moderation were fine. At times I found it easier just to stick to rules about food, like no animal products (my vegan phase), or no carbs (my drastic "control diabetes" phase). I have gone from having no energy despite plenty of sleep to waking up ready to go and staying like that all day. I doubled over in stomach pain at two different times in my life but now never have stomach discomfort at all. I have gone from not being able to be around animals or go for a run without having an asthma attack to enjoying soccer and pets again. Most importantly, I have gone from stressing about the damage type 1 diabetes is doing to my body to being confident that I am preventing a large portion of the damage that could come from the disease. All of these things were accomplished by taking the steps outlined in Chapter 16.

These transformations were not easy. Sometimes it is hard for people to understand why I am so confident that this approach can work for them too, but that's because they don't know all the work that has gone into my recommendations. Over the years I have learned so much and will continue to do so. I have found that my health, nutrition, and medical educations have been good but fell far short of truly enabling me to achieve health for myself and my patients. Luckily, my obsession has kept me gaining information through reading research and health-focused books, listening to podcasts, and attending conferences.

I'll never forget when things really dawned on me though. It was my first year in chiropractic school. I had come a long way as far as my health was concerned but there were still times when I would get symptoms. During one of these times I remember having to leave class and go and lay on the couch in the lobby because I was having gastrointestinal pain. It was so bad that it was causing back pain. Despite the pain, I remember thinking how we had learned in one class or another how viscera (internal organs) can cause (somatic) muscle pain. It was called viscerosomatic pain.

I don't recall the specific thought trail in my head but I eventually got to thinking about how in class we had learned about our bodies' ability to adapt to different situations by way of our autonomic nervous system. I felt my stomach pain again and thought to myself that for whatever reason my body was not adapting very well to whatever was going on. Some kind of light bulb went off. I started asking myself why my body was not adapting well to whatever was causing my pain. I told myself that maybe it didn't know how to adapt to whatever it was experiencing (I would later find out that it was poor diet choices). I had no idea where to start but I was now asking the right question. What was my body encountering that it was not built to adapt to?

As I found the answers to that question, over the following years I saw monumental increases in my personal health. It was all the proof I needed to know that the recommendations in Chapter 16 work. But through the years I have found proof that those recommendations work for many, many others as well.

Chapter 18: Proof

"To ward off disease or recover health, people as a rule find it easier to depend on healers than to attempt the more difficult task of living wisely."

-Rene Dubos

When I was backpacking through Central America I came across a book that would end up being my all-time favorite book. It is written by Michael Crichton—yes, the guy who wrote *Jurassic Park*. Most people don't know that Crichton went to medical school before he decided to become a writer. The book I came across was his nonfiction book, *Travels,* and in it he discusses some of his thoughts on the perplexing world of medicine. Within this discussion he said something that has stuck with me to this day:

> I had already concluded that the best way to think about disease was to imagine that you caused It. Maybe that was literally true, and maybe it wasn't. The point was that the best strategy in dealing with your illness was to act as if you had control over it, and could change its course. That enabled you to stay in charge of your own life.

I don't think that Crichton really thought we cause all of our diseases. Rather, he is just stating his opinion about the best mental strategy to dealing with disease. But when I read this, I was halfway through my medical education, and I think it stuck with me because deep down I knew that what was a mental trick for Crichton was in fact reality. The vast majority of the diseases we suffer from are caused—even if unintentionally—by how we have chosen to live our lives as a society. The silver lining is that this also means we do, in fact, have control over our lives when it comes to disease.

I have claimed a lot of things in this book so far. I have claimed that the Western medical system is failing. I have claimed that the reason we are experiencing such poor health is because we are suffering from the effects of a massive, evolutionarily quick, self-inflicted environment and lifestyle change. I have claimed that we may even be interrupting our process of evolution, causing us to devolve. I have claimed that by changing our personal environment though lifestyle change we can have profound effects on health and reverse many chronic diseases. If you have doubt in any of these claims then good for you—doubt is healthy! Doubt in the practices of Medical Inc. is what led me to begin my own quest for what truly creates health. Whatever sparks doubt in you, I urge you to go and look into that topic yourself or make the changes I suggested in the previous chapter and pay attention to the results.

If someone came to me tomorrow and showed me evidence that all, or part, of what I have said was untrue, I would take that information into account. However, it would probably not change my overall approach to the patients I coach back to health. Academic and scientific arguments pale in comparison to the results I see with real people every single day. If what I do ever stops working or I find more effective ways to get results for my patients, then, and only then, would I change my approach to health coaching and medicine. Willingness to change is how science advances, but I haven't found anything that works near as well as what I present in Chapter 16. We have to remember that the best evidence is not the evidence gathered in randomized controlled trials done on other people but the evidence your body gives you every single day. If you truly feel great and have no health issues whatsoever, then you are living a life compatible with health or you have really hardy genes. If you have even a slight complaint, there is probably an explanation, and that explanation is probably something you can address with changes to your environment. The best approach is not to see how a group of other people in a research study responded to treatment; it is to look into your personal environment and see what you can change to alter your body's response to the world.

Many, many practitioners, including functional medicine doctors, naturopaths, and knowledgeable health coaches get outstanding results with their patients and clients, but you won't find them documented in the journals of Western medicine. The reason they have never been documented in the medical journals is because those results did not happen within Western medicine's walls or through means Western medicine deems valid.

What's also important to note is that even if revolutionary research is completed in a research lab today, it would take about 17 years for that to end up being advice that your doctor gives you on your next visit.[1] The process of new research turning into medical teaching material and then turning into medical advice to patients is a long one, and it is more political than scientific. We cannot sit and wait for the answer to our health problems to appear sometime in the future. We have to look to the past and use what we know to construct a new personal environment that allows us to thrive. Moving your personal environment more in line with the environment we evolved in for millions of years is the only way to achieve radiant health.

To be sure, I do not completely write off research and medical treatments, which can also be useful in creating a healthier personal environment. It's just that the best methods are typically not utilized in a traditional doctor's office.

There are scientists who are truly passionate about figuring out how the body works and what we can do to make it work optimally. One of these people is physician and researcher Dr. Zach Bush. Through scientific research he has shown that losing contact with the elements of nature—certain molecules in dirt in this case—have literally left the cells in our bodies with an inability to connect and communicate.[2] His work has even brought into question every bit of medical research that has ever been done in a sterile Petri dish, because the conditions of a sterile Petri dish are not the conditions of the body. It turns out that dirt and bacteria are just as important for our physiology as the vitamins and minerals studied in biochemistry. How well can we really say we understand the body when we haven't studied it in the proper conditions?

Dr. Bush's work, and the work of many others, will continue to show us the best ways to return our body to the most natural environment possible within the confines of our modern world. In the meantime, we should immerse ourselves in the ancient wisdom of our natural world—that not-so-sterile environment—in order to achieve health, rather than heavily relying on a broken, profit-driven system. Remaining grounded in that natural wisdom and taking advantage of the least harmful modern approaches when necessary is the "best of both worlds" approach to our health epidemic.

For further proof of the wisdom of a more natural way of life, we can look at the work of Weston Price. Weston Price was a dentist, who for many summers in the 1930s traveled all over the world to find and study groups of people who were living more traditional lifestyles, or even hunter-gatherer lifestyles, and therefore, had been least affected by Western society. He visited 12 different isolated groups of traditional societies that varied from isolated Gaelic people in the British Isles to Eskimos in North America, to tribes in Africa, to various peoples throughout the pacific islands and Australia. What he found was amazing.

Dr. Price was a dentist, so he was mainly interested in why these groups of people had very little incidence of tooth decay, even without Western hygiene practices, and why they had perfectly formed dental arches. What he observed is that each group he studied ate a nutrient-rich diet. Each diet had specific, almost sacred, foods, which most of the time included some sort of fat, mostly animal fat. These people would go to great lengths to ensure that they had the quality food they knew would keep them healthy. Women and men who were set to marry would follow special diets even higher in these nutrient-dense foods months before their marriage, because they understood the increased need for nutrition it takes to conceive and produce a healthy baby. In order to survive, these people had to be sure their bodies received high amounts of nutrition so that they would function at the highest level. In modern society we have made life so "easy" that we don't need to get as much nutrition to ensure survival. This has led to declining health, much like we see in organic versus conventional produce. Organic produce has more nutrients, because it needs those nutrients to survive—we have not made their lives so easy by killing all the weeds and pests around them.

Aside from outstanding teeth and dental arches, Dr. Price also found that these people had little or no incidence of common chronic diseases such as diabetes, heart disease, cancer, or mental disorders.[3] Their elders were still very healthy, able to keep up with and perform the same tasks that younger members could, and very rarely became a burden to society by needing caretakers. In these groups of people, the lack of chronic disease and prevalence of healthy aging was a result of living closer to the environment that comes natural to humans. For the whole of their lives they were eating plentiful wild foods and using their bodies in natural ways in order to get it. They also lived far from the industrial and capitalist modern world and therefore had less toxicants and stress to deal with. Turns out this way of life is much more compatible with health.

What is even more interesting is that as Western culture and food started to appear in close proximity to these groups of people, those of them who decided to leave and eat a Western diet of processed foods experienced a significant drop in health. This wasn't over generations either; it happened immediately. He even had an example of identical twins where one had decided to stay in the traditional society and live the traditional way and the other had gone into the Western world and starting eating a Western diet. The difference in health of these two individuals with identical genes was eye opening. Through Dr. Price's work it is clear that the people living similarly to our ancient ancestors were masters of their health, even without the use of modern nutritional information, medical research, and modern medicine. Unfortunately, Dr. Price's work was largely ignored by the medical and dental communities and remains so to this day. A copy of his book, *Nutrition and Physical Degeneration,* is a must read for any health enthusiast.

In his book, *The World Until Yesterday,* Jared Diamond talks about finding similar phenomena while observing different populations on New Guinea beginning in 1964. He noticed that they did not suffer from the diseases that plague Western society like diabetes, cardiovascular disease, and cancers. He also noticed that they were extremely fit. They were able to carry heavy loads or hike up mountains quickly and with ease. Back then many New Guineans had not adopted a Western diet. Diamond says that 90% of their calories came from the crops sweet potato, taro, and yams, though they still ate wild animals. Obviously this suggests that it is possible to achieve better health from farming, but I would like to point out that sweet potato, taro, and yams have far more nutritional value than the crops that make up the majority of calories in the Western diet (corn, wheat, and soy). As far as diet goes, this shows that it is not so much about the watching how many fats, carbs, and proteins you consume but more about focusing on the nutrient richness of those macronutrients. As I have said previously, we live in a binary society where we like to label something as either good or bad and argue about it. We like to place blame on one macronutrient or another and totally demonize it when what really matters is the nutrient density and processing of our food.

We also have to realize that these New Guineans were not exposed to many—or perhaps any—of the toxins that have shown up in the Western world. They were natural births and breastfed with no overuse of antibiotics, which creates highly functioning immune and digestive systems. They lived in a natural light cycle, and definitely didn't have exposure to EMFs. Although they were not full-blown hunter-gatherers, they were living lives much closer to those of our ancient ancestors. Diamond's observational research provides yet more evidence that a change in lifestyle is what will lead us to health.

I believe our bodies are still set up for a hunter-gatherer lifestyle; however, the populations that Weston Price and Jared Diamond have observed show us that better health is clearly achievable without going all the way back to living in small, mobile hunter-gatherer groups out in the wild. We just need to start taking little steps to move back in that direction. Even if the government and researchers don't believe these observations hold any merit, you would think they would at least stimulate their curiosity and that, for the sake of humanity, they would spend a little more time and money looking into these populations to find out why they have such great health outcomes. Sadly, they haven't done this, most likely because the medical model is about profit and spending money on this type of research is not likely to produce results that they can use to bring revenue to Medical Inc.

Lastly, my most convincing proof is the results that I have seen with the people that I coach back to health. I have guided numerous people in their efforts to achieve higher levels of health through modifying the environment around them. For example, about three years ago a 44-year-old man came to me wanting to see what he could do about his type 2 diabetes, high blood pressure, liver disease, and rheumatoid arthritis (RA). He had to call in sick to work when his RA was bad and he was missing out on Boy Scout trips with his son. After an initial consultation and assessment, he and his wife determined that they could make some diet changes in their family. I constructed a diet and food grade supplement plan that would address his specific issues, and after three weeks of adherence to the plan, he and his prescribing doctor decided he could go without his diabetic medication. After eight weeks he was weaned off of his blood pressure medication because his doctor said his blood pressure was dropping too low. After twelve weeks his liver tests came back normal for the first time in ten years. His doctor was astounded. At this point his RA flare-ups had decreased dramatically. In those first three months his wife lost twenty-five pounds while following the plan with him. This was all just from changing diet. Over the last two years they have made other changes in movement routines, and have started to reduce their exposure to the toxins they didn't even know they were coming in contact with. Today he and his family are happy and healthy, and the last time I talked to them his daughter told me that she could not believe the change she has seen in her father.

As another example, a little over a year ago a twenty-three-year-old woman came to me for help with her long term depression, food and environmental allergies, weekly migraines, and chronic pain. She was on anti-depressants, painkillers, and was taking allergy shots. She was struggling to find the energy to get through the day and would often get colds that would last for two weeks, which was making work as a nurse difficult. We determined that a gut healing protocol was the best route for her. She agreed to follow a diet that promotes gut healing and to take food grade supplements known for healing the gut. Upon checking in with her after three weeks she reported that she had not seen much change in her main symptoms, but she said that she did have more energy. She said the diet was easy to follow and that it wouldn't be a problem to continue. After six weeks she felt that she no longer needed the painkillers and hadn't had a migraine in a few weeks. After three months she felt great, and I sent her to a doctor in her area to wean her off her anti-depressant. I put together an exercise program for her because she felt like she now had the energy. She did struggle over the next few months because anti-depressants are hard to wean patients from due to the changes they cause in the brain. However, since we had laid a healthy foundation, in time she was able to completely stop taking the anti-depressant. The last time I talked to her I asked her about her allergies and she told me that she had forgotten they had even been one of her complaints, because they hadn't been bothering her.

This is the power of slowing our environmental change and restoring proper expression of your genes. The greatest result I get with my patients is not the reversing of diabetes, the weight loss, or the elimination of symptoms, it is the high satisfaction that they seem to get when they gain back control of their health by means of their own hard work. They find it empowering to know that when it comes to health, they do not have to be so dependent on healthcare professionals all the time. If they educate themselves and take control of their lifestyles, then health becomes something that they create for themselves, not something they hope to find at a doctor's office.

Ancient humans spent their entire lives doing things that would make them healthy enough to be able to reproduce and keep their offspring safe until adulthood. They constantly looked for food, water, warmth, and shelter. Nowadays we spend our whole day at a job so that we can make money, which forces health creation to take a back seat; honestly, it may even be in the trunk. But how are you supposed to find the time to live in a way that creates health and make the money you need to function in society?

One step at a time. With each step you will become more empowered, gain confidence, and get closer to the health you deserve. With each step we take to create individual health, we as a species will get closer and closer to halting the rapid, unhealthy, and unsustainable changes taking place on the planet we call home.

Epilogue

"If you ever start taking things too seriously, just remember we are talking monkeys on an organic spaceship flying through the universe."

—Joe Rogan

Health is not a gift; it cannot be given by a doctor, by your genes, or any god. Health is also not an exact state. Rather, health is a dynamic that has been driven by ecology and evolution since the beginning of life as we know it here on Earth. Health is when equilibrium exists between the biology of any living thing and the ecology of the world it inhabits. To be "healthy," we must take strides to balance this equilibrium. To achieve your personal best health, learn about the environment your genes hold their roots in and become a master of the interaction between your genes and your environment.

In defiance of the nature laws of the world, we have taken species of plants out of the wild and have made their life easy through the use of pesticides and herbicides for the sake of increasing their yields, and we have bred wild animals in captivity so that they are never exposed to the dangers of the wild and are always provided with enough food. These situations have resulted in weaker species of plants and animals because over time those species have lost the ability to survive in a wild environment. Likewise, we humans who have so quickly taken ourselves out of our natural environment, away from our natural stressors, have become a weaker species. All life is driven by the struggle to overcome stress-inducing obstacles to survive and pass on genes. Replacing our natural obstacles with unnatural stressors has weakened humans and created our epidemic of chronic disease. In the long run, if we choose to stay on this path, we should not expect to survive as a species.

As Dian Fossey says, "One of the basic steps in saving a threatened species is to learn about it: its diet, its mating and reproductive process, its range patterns, its social behavior." We are the most successful species on the planet, so we are not quite in need of saving yet; however, we are far behind on understanding this important information about ourselves. Many of us think we know a lot about the behavior of humans, but we tend only to know how post-Agricultural Revolution humans—humans in captivity, so to speak—eat, mate, travel, and socialize. Generally speaking, we don't know much about how humans behaved in the natural world we are adapted to. I would conjecture that if we began to use the knowledge we do have about how humans once lived, we may stumble upon the information required for saving our own species.

Saving our species has become an intellectual matter as well as an obeying-the-laws-of-nature-and-evolution matter. We need to think and cooperate our way out of our situation while also realizing that life is about struggle for survival, and that Earth was never intended to be a utopia. I cannot help using one last Rene Dubos quote here:

Man cannot hope to find another paradise on Earth, because paradise is a static concept while human life is a dynamic process. Man could escape danger only by renouncing adventure, by abandoning that which has given to the human condition its unique character and genius among the rest of living things. Since the days of the cave man, the earth has never been a Garden of Eden, but a Valley of Decision where resilience is essential to survival. The earth is not a resting place. Man has elected to fight, not necessarily for himself, but for a process of emotional, intellectual, and ethical growth that goes on forever. To grow in the midst of dangers is the fate of the human race, because it is the law of the spirit.

One of the "dangers" that Dubos speaks of is the health epidemic we are facing. As he says, we must "grow in the midst of it." It's true that survival includes struggle, though the chronic diseases we suffer from are an unnecessary part of our modern day struggle. I often daydream about what I call my romanticized state of the world. This romanticized state is one where everyone is not so focused on being successful in our capitalist society and instead puts their health and well-being first and foremost. If it was possible to conduct experiments on this romanticized view in a lab you can bet I would be attempting to get it done. Since it is not possible to do in a lab, we have to hope that it starts to happen within society. Could you imagine if things like refined sugars, refined grains, oxidized fats, chemical toxins, heavy metals, and unnatural stress didn't exist? No? Okay, maybe it's just me who daydreams about things like that! Regardless, if those things did not exist, I hypothesize that, on a global scale, humans would experience much greater levels of physical and mental health. I also hypothesize that it would result in less crime, less spending on healthcare, less destruction of our environment, and a society that would come together and solve the problems that face us in the future. I hope one day to see my daydream become a reality.

When thinking about the problems we face as a species, we tend to think of things such as our epidemic of chronic disease, the extinction of more and more species, the pollution of our environment, and the economic inequality between populations as problems. They are not the problem; they are the symptoms. They are the symptoms of us living separately from the natural world that we evolved in for millions of years. Just like Western medical doctors are trained to identify and treat the symptoms of humans in an unnatural world instead of finding the root causes, we as a society are identifying the symptoms of a very successful species living outside of its natural world and frantically trying to correct the symptoms rather than fix the problem. I believe that a good first step to addressing the problem is for each of us individually to take steps that move us back toward our natural environment.

I realize that this is not always an easy task, and when I lecture to groups or work with people to change their health, many people make the mistake of assuming that they cannot possibly make the changes I am suggesting because either their day-to-day lives would not allow it or they think that it is impossible for them to give up the "pleasures" that many unhealthy habits in today's world offer. In a way they are right—the society we have created has made it very hard to work a full time job and raise a family as well as do all that is needed to achieve optimal health. To tackle this hurdle, as well as mental hurdles, we have to get back to thinking in line with the philosophical perspective mentioned all the way back in the beginning of this book. We have to frame our question a little differently. Nora Gedgaudas says it best:

Is living about getting a brief high from a fleeting indulgence, or is it about enjoying ongoing energy, clarity, and real symptom-free health because you made consistent, quality choices that actually support the health of your body and brain? And when it comes to the catchphrase 'everything in moderation,' by what (or whose) standard might the term moderation be defined...or rationalized? Who today can afford (much less enjoy) 'moderate' inflammation, endocrine disruption, health, immune dysfunction, or health compromise?

We may feel that it is impossible to live in a way that achieves health while also fulfilling the responsibilities that society demands of us, but in the end, if we fail to achieve health then eventually we won't be able to fulfill those responsibilities anyway. To be fair, it is not only our individual lives and decisions that are keeping us from making the change, it is also the high expectations of the society we live in, which make it very hard to achieve our health goals. But when faced with the unrealistic expectations of society, we are more likely to conquer those expectations with a body running on all cylinders instead of a body that is chronically weakened. Surviving in the world used to be solely about finding the resources you needed to thrive in order to ensure survival and gene transmission. Today life is about gaining one resource—money—in order to buy other resources. Unfortunately, through this way of life, we have lost the knowledge of what creates health and we don't even know what to buy with the money we earn in order to ensure optimal health and the transmission of our best genes.

If we want to make changes in our individual health, the health of the environment, and the future of our species, then each of us individually has to create the world around us that we want to live in rather than accepting the environment that society has created. If everyone was a little more selfish (sounds funny, doesn't it?) and started making positive health changes in their personal lives, and their families' lives, then I predict the hard situations that our species will face in the future will be easier to find solutions for. By doing things that will create less of a negative impact on our bodies we will also have less of a negative impact on our planet, because the environment that surrounds our bodies is the same environment that is our planet.

I do realize that if everyone in the world decided tomorrow to make the changes I suggest in this book then it is quite possible that at first we would have more problems than we would fix. Problems would arise, as the shift of consumers' desires would alter the economic system we have in place, but I believe that those problems would be much easier solved than the ones that are at the end of the path we are on. I would much rather be faced with the problem of how to ensure that everyone has access high quality, nutrient dense, organic food than the problem of growing food when our soil can no longer support life because they have been destroyed by unsustainable agricultural practices. Our modern way of life has created so many health concerns like this that those concerns are distracting from our ability to come together and focus on other societal issues like socioeconomic inequality and racism.

Humankind seems to believe in the illusion that if we just give technology time, eventually it will create a world of health and ease for us. I feel this line of thinking will lead to a tragic ending. I am reminded of the movie, *Elysium*, in which a medical machine can eradicate all traces of disease in a patient almost instantaneously. When I first saw this I dismissed it as an outlandish but great device for a science fiction movie. However, after adding to my practice some of the newer healing technologies like Frequency Specific

Microcurrent, Pulse Electromagnetic Frequency, and Infrared Light Therapy, I am forced to think that a machine like this may one day be a reality.

I don't think machines like this would be beneficial, however. These machines would only further allow us to save ourselves while simultaneously destroying our world, until eventually we could not survive without machines. Would a new species of man-machine arrive? Maybe. Perhaps humans would just evolve into something else. But I believe any scenario which allows our environment to be corrupted while preserving ourselves comes back to bite us in the end, when we lack the natural resources required to keep ourselves alive. The more logical approach lies with us continuing to progress with one foot while the other is planted firmly in the wisdom of our past. If someone alive today wants health this is what must be done.

The last essential concept needed to ensure that we are successful at turning the fate of humans around is that we are going to have to do it as a connected and unified community. Believe it or not, this is also a selfish solution. Dr. Zach Bush, the physician and researcher mentioned earlier, has found that when cellular connections and communications become damaged then cells start to behave differently compared to when they are able to easily communicate with their neighboring cells. When isolated, cells behave in ways that are very damaging to neighboring cells and the body as a whole; they act as if they are the only one in the community and do things that are best for themselves and not the community. When this happens it ultimately drives chronic disease on a systemic level. Unfortunately, we see a parallel in isolation among humans today. While the internet has connected us in many ways it has also driven us away from human contact and true human connection. Individuals who become socially isolated and distant many times become dysfunctional within our society; some even end up lashing out. It makes you wonder if there is any correlation to someone having dysfunction at the cellular level and that cellular behavior manifesting itself in behaviors of an individual. Even Dubos knew that the real measure of health is the "ability of the individual to function in a manner acceptable to himself and to the group of which he is a part."

Just like our cells function better when they can effectively connect and communicate with each other, so do we humans. The solutions I present in this book are going to take effort, and the more we connect as supportive communities the better chance we are going to have. One of my favorite quotes is by Howard Thurman. He says, "Don't ask what the world needs. Ask what makes you come alive, and go do it. Because what the world needs is people who have come alive." Only by coming alive through following our passions and connecting with one another will we overcome our health epidemic and ensure a healthy future for our species.

Acknowledgements

There are many people to thank but there are three I want to specifically mention here.

First is Kevin Stone, who after hearing me ramble on about health was the one who suggested that I write it down and kept subtly reminding me to do it until I did.

Second is April Bacon, my editor. Her suggestions and critiques were so valuable in this process.

Lastly, I want to thank Kinga, my wife. Aside from her support I could also count on her to say, "I don't believe you" when I read her something from the book she didn't like. Any area in the book where I go a little farther to make my point is thanks to the "Kinga effect."

Appendix I –Further Readings and Documentaries

Prologue

1. *Dr. Bernstein's Diabetes Solution* – Richard K. Bernstein, MD

2. Unofficial College Transcript, the University of North Carolina Asheville – Stephen Hussey (Fall 2005-Spring 2009)

3. *SOAR Study Skills: A Simple and Efficient System for Getting Better Grades in Less Time* – Susan Kruger

Chapter 2

1. *The Disease Delusion* – Jeffrey Bland, PhD

2. Fed Up (documentary)

3. Hungry for Change (documentary)

Chapter 4

1. Bought (documentary)

2. The Greater Good (documentary)

3. *Overdosed America* – John Abramson

4. *A Mind of Your Own* – Kelly Brogan, MD

5. *Rockefeller Medicine Men: Medicine and Capitalism in America* – E. Richard Brown and Donald E. Johnson

6. *Bad Science* – Ben Goldacre, MD

7. *The Structure of Scientific Revolutions* – Thomas Khun

8. Doctored (documentary)

Chapter 6

1. *On the Origins of Species* – Charles Darwin

2. *The Greatest Show on Earth* – Richard Dawkins

Chapter 8

1. *A Brief History of Nearly Everything* – Bill Bryson

2. *The Third Chimpanzee* – Jared Diamond

3. *Why Nations Fail* – Daron Acemoglu and James A. Robinson

4. *Sapiens* – Yuval Noah Harari

5. *Food Forensics* – Mike Adams

Chapter 10

1. *Guns, Germs, and Steel* – Jared Diamond

2. *The Biology of Belief: Unleashing the Power of Consciousness, Matter & Miracles* – Bruce Lipton

3. *The Epigenetics Revolution: How Modern Biology is Rewriting Our Understanding of Genetics, Disease, and Inheritance* – Nessa Carey

4. *The World Until Yesterday* – Jared Diamond

Chapter 12

1. *The Sixth Extinction* – Elizabeth Kolbert

2. *Collapse* – Jared Diamond

Chapter 14

1. *The Selfish Gene* – Richard Dawkins

Chapter 16

Food

1. *Eat Fat, Get Thin* – Mark Hyman, MD

2. *The Great Cholesterol Myth: Why Lowing Cholesterol Won't Prevent Heart Disease-and the Statin-Free Plan that Will* – Johnny Bowden

3. *Deep Nutrition* – Cate Shanahan, MD

4. *The Bulletproof Diet* – Dave Asprey

5. *Primal Fat Burner* – Nora Gedgaudas

6. *The Fourfold Path to Healing* – Thomas Cowan, MD and Sally Fallon

7. *Edible Wild Plants: A North American Field Guide to Over 200 Natural Foods* – Thomas Elias and Peter Dykeman

8. *The Omnivore's Dilemma* – Michael Pollan

9. *The Botany of Desire* – Michael Pollan

Toxicants

1. *Clean, Green, and Lean* – Walter Crinnion, ND

2. *Food Forensics* – Mike Adams

3. *Genetic Roulette: The Documented Health Risks of Genetically Engineered Foods* – Jeffrey M. Smith

Water

1. *The Fourth Phase of Water* – Gerald Pollack, PhD

2. *Healing Waters: The Ultimate Guide to Taking the Waters* – Nathaniel Altman

Gut Healing

1. *The Skinny Gut Diet* – Brenda Watson

2. *Brain Maker* – David Perlmutter, MD

Movement

1. *Move Your DNA* – Katy Bowman

2. *Movement Matters* – Katy Bowman

3. *Anatomy Trains: Myofascial Meridians for Manual and Movement Therapists* – Thomas Myers

4. *Functional Training Handbook* – Craig Liebenson, DC

Stress

1. *Why Zebras Don't Get Ulcers* – Robert Sapolsky, PhD

2. *Human Heart, Cosmic Heart* – Thomas Cowan, MD

3. *Minimalism – Live a Meaningful Life* – Joshua Fields Millburn and Ryan Nicodemus

4. *The More Beautiful World Our Hearts Know is Possible* – Charles Eisenstein

Spirituality
1. *The Seven Spiritual Laws of Success: A Practical Guide to the Fulfillment of Your Dreams* – Deepak Chopra, MD
2. *Molecules of Emotion* – Candace Pert, PhD
3. *The Varieties of Religious Experience* – William James

Dentistry
1. *Toxic Dentistry Exposed* –Graeme Munro-Hall, BDS and Lilian Munro-Hall
2. *Nutrition and Physical Degeneration* – Weston Price, DDS
3. *Holistic Dental Care – The Complete Guide to Healthy Teeth and Gums* – Nadine Artemis and Victor Zeines, DDS

Chapter 18
1. *Travels* – Michael Crichton

Appendix II – Resources

Health Coaching

1. www.resourceyourhealth.com – Our headquarters for health coaching, our menu service, and other resources for achieving health. This is where potential clients can contact me.

Organizations

1. Hunt Gather Grow Foundation – Excellent resource for bringing aspects of our ancient ancestors lifestyle into our own.
2. The Institute for Responsible Technology – Great resource for anyone looking for information about genetically modified organisms (GMO's). Lots of information and science to explore here.
3. Weston A. Price Foundation – Foundation that supports people in their quest to find food that creates health. It is largely based on the work of Weston Price.
4. The Savory Institute – Institute dedicated to restoring the quality of our land through responsible, sustainable, and health promoting animal agricultural practices.
5. THINCS: The international Network of Cholesterol Skeptics – Organization of doctors and scientists who recognize that our current approach to medicine is not adequate and work to blend

modern medicine and research with health promoting lifestyle practices.

Health Podcasts

1. Oneradionetwork.com – Daily shows with Patrick Timpone that talk about health, wealth, and well-being.
2. Bulletproof Radio – Biohacker Dave Asprey interviews guests about the best ways to achieve health in the modern world.
3. Rewild Yourself Podcast – Danial Vitalis discusses how best to rewild yourself through interviews and informational episodes.
4. Katy Says – Biomechanist Katy Bowman discusses natural movement.
5. Revolution Health Radio – Chris Kresser discusses health and strategies to address common chronic illnesses.
6. Primal Body Primal Mind Radio – Nora Gedgaudas discusses, promotes, and strategizes about primal practices.
7. The Doctors Farmacy – Dr. Mark Hyman interviews top doctors, researchers, and journalists in the areas of health and food policy.

High Quality Meat

1. Eatwild.com – Find farmers near you who are raising and selling grass-fed and pastured meats.
2. US Wellness Meats (www.grasslandmeat.com) - Grass-fed and pastured meats delivered right to your door.
3. Butcherbox.com – Grass-fed and pastured meats delivered right to your door.

Water

1. Findaspring.com – Find out if there is a natural spring in your area.
2. AquaTru – The best countertop water filter on the market.
3. Big Berkey – The best large quantity gravity powered water filters on the market.

Supplements

1. Radiantlifecatalog.com

2. Surthrival.com

3. Naturalnews.com – Go to the store and know that all the supplements have been lab tested for verification and confirmation of low toxicity.

Miscellaneous

1. Cultures for Health – Your source for all the materials and information to start making your own fermented foods.

2. Sprouthouse.com – Your source for all the materials and information you need to start sprouting.

3. Infrared Saunas – Very useful for detoxification, building 4th phase water, and putting you into a parasympathetic state. Sunlighten has the best saunas on the market.

4. Living Libations – Excellent source for non-toxic beauty care products for men and women.

Notes

Prologue

1. Accurso A, Bernstein RK, Dahlqvist A, Draznin B, et al. "Dietary Carbohydrate restriction in type 2 diabetes mellitus and metabolic syndrome: Time for a critical appraisal." Nutr Metabol (2008); 5: 9.

2. L. Z. Agudelo et al., Skeletal Muscle PGC-1α1 Modulates Kynurenine Metabolism and Mediates Resilience to Stress-induced Depression, *Cell* 159, no. 1 (September 25, 2014): 33-45

Chapter 2

1. Max Roser (2017) – 'Life Expectancy'. *Published online at OurWorldInData.org.* Retrieved from: https://ourworldindata.org/life-expectancy/ [Online Resource]

2. Tackling the burden of chronic diseases in the USA. Lancet 2009; 373(9659):185. Accessed at http://www.thelancet.com/journals/lancet/article/PIIS0140-6736(09)60048-9/fulltext

3. S. Jay Olshansky, Ph.D., Douglas J. Passaro, M.D., et al. "A Potential Decline in Life Expectancy in the United States in the 21st Century". N Engl J Med 2005; 352:1138-1145 March 17, 2005 DOI: 10.1056/NEJMsr043743

4. Davis, K., & Commonwealth Fund. (2014). *Mirror, mirror on the wall: How the performance of the U.S. health care system compares internationally: 2014 update*. New York, NY: Commonwealth Fund.

Chapter 4

1. Himmelstein, D. U., MD, Thorne, D., PhD, Warren, E., JD, & Woolhandler, S., MD, MPH. (2009). Medical Bankruptcy in the United States, 2007; Results of a National Study. *The American Journal of Medicine, 122*(8), 741-746.

2. Leonard, W. R., Sorensen, M. V., Galloway, V. A., Spencer, G. J., Mosher, M., Osipova, L., & Spitsyn, V. A. (2002). Climatic influences on basal metabolic rates among circumpolar populations. *American Journal of Human Biology, 14*(5), 609-620. doi:10.1002/ajhb.10072

3. Leonard, W. R., Snodgrass, J. J., & Sorensen, M. V. (2005). METABOLIC ADAPTATION IN INDIGENOUS SIBERIAN POPULATIONS. *Annual Review of Anthropology, 34*(1), 451-471. doi:10.1146/annurev.anthro.34.081804.120558

Chapter 8

1. Kitahara, T., Koyama, N., Matsuda, J., Aoyama, Y., Hirakata, Y., Kamihira, S. et al. Antimicrobial activity of saturated fatty acids and fatty amines against methicillin-resistant *Staphylococcus aureus*. *Biol Pharm Bull*. 2004; 27: 1321–1326

2. Feldlaufer, M. F., Knox, D. A., Lusby, W. R., & Shimanuki, H. (1993). Antimicrobial activity of fatty acids against Bacillus larvae, the causative agent of American foulbrood disease. *Apidologie, 24*(2), 95-99. doi:10.1051/apido:19930202

3. Hawks, John. Selections for smaller brains in Holocene human evolution. Department of Anthropology, University of Wisconsin—Madison. 28 Feb 2011.

4. Ryan, T. M., & Shaw, C. N. (2015). Gracility of the modern Homo sapiens skeleton is the result of decreased biomechanical loading. *PNAS,112*(2), 372-377. doi:10.1073/pnas.1418646112

Chapter 10

1. Mills, Dora Anne. "Chronic Disease: The Epidemic of the Twentieth Century." Maine Policy Review 9.1 (2000): 50 -65, https://digitalcommons.library.umaine.edu/mpr/vol9/iss1/8.

2. Lipton, B. H., Bensch, K. G., & Karasek, M. A. (march 1991). Microvessel endothelial cell transdifferentiation: phenotypic characterization. *Differentiation,46*(2), 117-133.

Chapter 12

1. Max Roser (2018)-"Fertility Rate". *Published online at OurWorldInData.org.* Retrieved from: 'https://ourworldindata.org/fertility-rate' [Online Resource]

2. Levine, H., Jorgensen, N., Martino-Andrade, A., Mendiola, J., Weksler-Derri, D., Mindlis, I., ... Swan, S. H. (2017). Temporal trends in sperm count: a systematic review and meta-regression analysis. *Human Reproduction Update*, 1-14. doi:10.1093/humupd/dmx022

3. Dwyer-Lindgren L, Bertozzi-Villa A, Stubbs RW, et al. Inequalities in Life Expectancy Among US Counties, 1980 to 2014Temporal Trends and Key Drivers. *JAMA Intern Med.* 2017; 177(7):1003–1011. doi:10.1001/jamainternmed.2017.0918

4. Birth Spacing and Risk of Adverse Perinatal Outcomes: a Meta-Analysis. (2006). *Obstetrics & Gynecology, 108*(1), 203. doi:10.1097/01.aog.0000226648.49888.53

Chapter 14

1. Smith JM. Survey Reports Improved Health After Avoiding Genetically Modified Foods. International Journal of Human Nutrition and Functional Medicine 2017; article in review

Chapter 16

1. The Pollution in Newborns: A Benchmark Investigation of Industrial Chemicals, Pollutants, and Pesticides in umbilical Cord Blood. (2005, July 14). Retrieved September 23, 2017, from

http://www.ewg.org/research/body-burden-pollution-newborns#.Wcb3-9SGM1I

2. Martin, J. A., Hamilton, B. E., Osterman, M. J., Driscoll, A. K., & Drake, P. (2018). Births: Final Data for 2016. *National Vital Statistics Report, 67*(1), 1-55. Retrieved from https://www.cdc.gov/nchs/data/nvsr/nvsr67/nvsr67_01.pdf

3. Duckett, S. K., Neel, J. P., Fontenot, J. P., & Clapham, W. M. (2009). Effects of winter stocker growth rate and finishing system on: III. Tissue proximate, fatty acid, vitamin, and cholesterol content 1. *Journal of Animal Science, 87*(9), 2961-2970. doi:10.2527/jas.2009-1850

4. Crinnion, Walter J. Organic foods contain higher levels of certain nutrients, lower levels of pesticides, and may provide health benefits for the consumer. *Alternative Medicine Review*, Apr. 2010, p. 4+. *Academic OneFile*, Accessed 28 Feb. 2017.

5. Di Angelantonio, E., Chowdhury, R., Forouhi, N. G., & Danesh, J. (2014). Association of Dietary, Circulating, and Supplement Fatty Acids With Coronary Risk. *Annals of Internal Medicine, 161*(6), 458. doi:10.7326/l14-5018-11

6. Cowan, T., MD. (2014). What Causes Heart Attacks. *Townsend Letter,*67-70.

7. Sharman, M. J., Kraemer, W. J., Love, D. M., Avery, N. G., Gomez, A. L., Scheett, T. P., & J. S. (2002). A Ketogenic Diet Favorably Affect Serum Biomarkers for Cardiovascular Disease in Normal-Weight Men. *Journal of Nutrition,132*(7), 1879-1885. Retrieved September 26, 2017, from http://jn.nutrition.org

8. Ravnskov, U., Diamond, D. M., Hama, R., Hamazaki, T., Hammarskjöld, B., Hynes, N., ... Sundberg, R. (2016). Lack of an association or an inverse association between low-density-lipoprotein cholesterol and mortality in the elderly: a systematic review. *BMJ Open, 6*(6), e010401. doi:10.1136/bmjopen-2015-010401

9. Chen, Q., Espey, M. G., Krishna, M. C., Mitchell, J. B., Corpe, C. P., Buettner, G. R., Levine, M. (2005). Pharmacologic ascorbic acid concentrations selectively kill cancer cells: Action as a pro-drug to deliver hydrogen peroxide to tissues. Proceeding of the National Academy of Sciences, 102(38), 13604-13609. Doi:10.1073/pnas.0506390102

10. Chen, P., Miah, M. R., & Aschner, M. (2016). Metals and Neurodegeneration. *F1000Research*, *5*, 366. doi:10.12688/f1000research.7431.1

11. Pupo, M., Pisano, A., Lappano, R., Santolla, M. F., De Francesco, E. M., Abonante, S., ... Maggiolini, M. (2012). Bisphenol A Induces Gene Expression Changes and Proliferative Effects through GPER in Breast Cancer Cells and Cancer-Associated Fibroblasts. *Environmental Health Perspectives*, *120*(8), 1177-1182. doi:10.1289/ehp.1104526

12. D.W. Laist, "Impacts of marine debris: entanglement of marine life in marine debris including a comprehensive list of species with entanglement and ingestion records," in Coe, J.M. Rogers, D.B. (eds), Marine Debris: Sources, Impacts, and Solutions: Springer-Verlag, New York, (1997) 99-139.

13. Nakamura, D., Yanagiba, Y., Duan, Z., Ito, Y., Okamura, A., Asaeda, N., ... Zhang, S. (2010). Bisphenol A may cause testosterone reduction by adversely affecting both testis and pituitary systems similar to estradiol. *Toxicology Letters*, *194*(1-2), 16-25. doi:10.1016/j.toxlet.2010.02.002

14. Shivarajashankara, Y.M., Shivashankara, A.R. (2012). Neurotoxic effects of Fluoride in endemic Skeletal Fluorosis and in Experimental Chronic Fluoride Toxicity. *Journal of Clinical and Diagnostic Research*, 6(4), 740-744.

15. Wagner, M., Oehlmann, J. (2009). Endocrine disruptors in bottled mineral water: total estrogenic burden and migration from

plastic bottles. *Environmental Science and Pollution Research*, 16(3), 278-286.

16. Marinelli, R., Feurst, B., Van der Zee, H., McGinn, A., & Marinelli, W. (1995). The Heart is not a Pump: A Refutation of the Pressure Propulsion Premise of Heart Function. *Frontier Perspectives*, 5(1).

17. Cryan, J.F., Dinan, T.G. (2012). Mind-altering microorganisms: the impact of the gut microbiota on brain and behavior. *Nature Reviews Neuroscience*, 13, 701-712.

18. Mullin, G. E., & Delzenne, N. M. (2014). The Human Gut Microbiome and Its Role in Obesity and the Metabolic Syndrome. *Integrative Weight Management*, 71-105. doi:10.1007/978-1-4939-0548-5_7

19. Huttenhower, C., Gevers, D., (2012). Structure, function and diversity of the healthy human microbiome. *Nature*, 486, 207-214.

20. Spector, T., & Leach, J. (2017, June 30). I spent three days as a hunter-gatherer to see if it would improve my gut health. Retrieved from http://theconversation.com/i-spent-three-days-as-a-hunter-gatherer-to-see-if-it-would-improve-my-gut-health-78773

21. Aiello, A. E., & Larson, E. (2003). Antibacterial cleaning and hygiene products as an emerging risk factor for antibiotic resistance in the community. *The Lancet Infectious Diseases*, 3(8), 501-506. doi:10.1016/s1473-3099(03)00723-0

22. Vighi, G., Marcucci, F., Sensi, L., Di Cara, G., & Frati, F. (2008). Allergy and the gastrointestinal system. *Clinical & Experimental Immunology*, 153, 3-6. doi:10.1111/j.1365-2249.2008.03713.x

23. Kalla, A., & Gosal, S. K. (2011). Effect of pesticide application on soil microorganisms. *Archives of Agronomy and Soil Science*, 57(6), 569-596. doi:10.1080/03650341003787582

24. Data from 2009, UNCCD. Securitizing the Ground, Grounding Security.

25. Bercik, P., Denou, E., Collins, J., Jackson, W., Lu, J., Jury, J., . . . Collins, S. (2011). The intestinal microbiota affect central levels of brain-derived neurotropic factor and behavior in mice. *Gastroenterology,141*, 599-609. doi:10.1053/j.gastro.2011.04.052.

26. Tillisch, K., Labus, J., Kilpatrick, L., Jiang, Z., Stains, J., Ebrat, B., . . Mayer, E. A. (2013). Consumption of Fermented Milk Product With Probiotic Modulates Brain Activity. *Gastroenterology,144*, 1394-1401.

27. Patil, H.R., MD, O'Keefe, J.H., MD, Lavie, C.J., MD, Magalski, A., MD, Vogel, R.A., MD, McCullough, P.A., MD. (2012). Cardiovascular Damage Resulting from Chronic Excessive Endurance Exercise. *Missouri Medicine*, 109(4), 312-321.

28. Hause M: "Pain and the nerve root." Spine 18(14):2053, (1993)

29. W. Kunert MD (1965) Functional Disorders of Internal Organs Due to Vertebral Lesions,CIBA Symposium 13 (3) :85-96

30. Rossi, W. A. (2001). Footwear: The primary cause of foot disorders. *Podiatry Management*, 129-138. Retrieved from https://www.correcttoes.com/foot-help/wp-content/uploads/2015/12/Rossi-FootwearTheprimarycauseofFootDisorders.pdf

31. Anagnostis, P., Athyros, V.G., Tziomalos, K., Karagiannis, A., Mikhalildis, D.P. (2009). The Pathogenic Role of Cortisol in the Metabolic Syndrome: A Hypothesis. *The Journal of Clinical Endocrinology & Metabolism*, 94(8), 2692-2701.

32. Baroldi, G., & Silver, M. D. (2004). *The Etiopathogenesis of Coronary Heart Disease: A Heretical Theory Based on Morphology* (2nd ed.). Georgetown, Texas: Eurekah.com/Landes Bioscience.

33. Scheer, F.A., Hilton, M.F., Mantzoros, C.S., Shea, S.A. (2009). Adverse Metabolic and Cardiovascular Consequences of Circadian

Misalignment. *Proceedings of the National Acadmey of Sciences of the United States of America*, 106(11), 4453-4458.

34. Roe, J.J., Thompson, C.W., Aspinall, P.A., Brewer, M.J., Duff, E.I, Miller, D., Clow, A. (2013). Green Space and Stress: Evidence from Cortisol Measures in Deprived Urban Communities. *International Journal of Environmental Research and Public Health*, 10(9), 4086-4103.

35. Czeisler, C. A., PhD, MD, Shanahan, T. L., BSc, Klerman, E. B., PhD, MD, Martens, H., MD, Brotman, D. J., A.B., Emens, J. S., BA, . . . Rizzo, J. F., MD. (1995). Suppression of Melatonin Secretion in Some Blind Patients by Exposure to Bright Light. *The New England Journal of Medicine,332*, 6-11. doi:DOI: 10.1056/NEJM199501053320102

36. Godley, B. F., Shamsi, F. A., Liang, F., Jarrett, S. G., Davies, S., & Boulton, M. (2005). Blue Light Induces Mitochondrial DNA Damage and Free Radical Production in Epithelial Cells. *Journal of Biological Chemistry*, *280*(22), 21061-21066. doi:10.1074/jbc.m502194200

37. Genuis, S.J. (2008) fielding a current idea: exploring the public health impact of electromagnetic radiation. Public Health, 122(2), 113-124.

38. Eger, H., Uwe Hagan, K., Lucas, B., Vogel, P., Voit, H. (2004). The Influence of Being Physically Near to a Cell Phone Transmission Mast on the Incidence of Cancer. *Umwelt·Medizin·Gesellschaft,* 17(4), 1-7. Retrieved from http://www.emf-health.com/PDFreports/Germanreport_celltower.pdf

39. Wolf, R., MD, Wolf, D., MD. (2004). Increased Incidence of Cancer Near a Cell Phone Transmitter Station. *International Journal of Cancer Prevention*, 1(2). Retrieved from http://www.emf-health.com/PDFreports/Israelstudy_celltower.pdf

40. Oberfeld, G. (2008). Environmental Epidemiological Study of Cancer Incidence in the Municipalities of Hausmannstätten & Vasoldsberg (Austria). Provincial Government of Styria, Department

8B, Provincial Public Health Office, Graz (Austria). Retrieved from http://www.emf-health.com/PDFreports/Austrianstudy.pdf

41. Pall, M. (2014). Microwave electromagnetic fields act by activating voltage-gated calcium channels: why the current international safety standards do not predict biological hazard. *Recent Research and Development in Cellular and Molecular Biology, 7*. Retrieved from http://www.electricalpollution.com/documents/Pallmicrow-vgccnoheat.pdf

42. Cheing, G. L., Li, X., Huang, L., Kwan, R. L., & Cheung, K. (2014). Pulsed electromagnetic fields (PEMF) promote early wound healing and myofibroblast proliferation in diabetic rats. *Bioelectromagnetics, 35*(3), 161-169. doi:10.1002/bem.21832

43. Esmail, M. Y., Sun, L., Yu, L., Xu, H., Shi, L., & Zhang, J. (2012). Effects of PEMF and glucocorticoids on proliferation and differentiation of osteoblasts. *Electromagnetic Biology and Medicine, 31*(4), 375-381. doi:10.3109/15368378.2012.662196

Chapter 18

1. Z. S. Morris, S. Woodring, and J. Grant, The Answer is 17 Years, What is the Question: Understanding Time Lags in Translational Research, *Journal of Royal Society of Medicine* 104, no. 12 (December 2011): 510-20

2. Gildea, J. J., Roberts, D. A., & Bush, Z. (2017). Protective Effects of Lignite Extract Supplement on Intestinal Barrier Function in Glyphosate-Mediated Tight Junction Injury. *Journal of Clinical Nutrition & Dietetics, 03*(01). doi:10.4172/2472-1921.100035

3. Price, W. A. (2016). *Nutrition and physical degeneration* (8th ed.). Lemon Grove, CA: Price-Pottenger.

About the Author

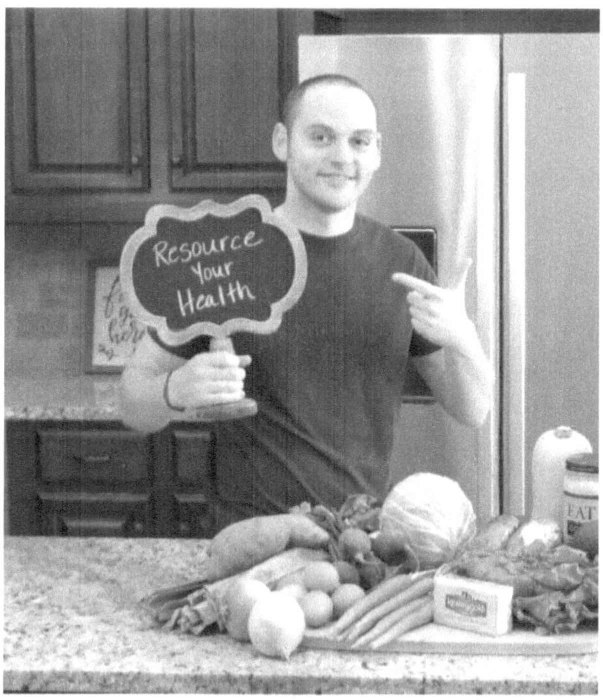

Dr. Stephen Hussey is a board certified Chiropractor and Functional Medicine practitioner. He has a bachelor's degree in health and wellness promotion from the University of North Carolina Asheville. He then went on to attend the University of Western States where he attained his Doctorate of Chiropractic and Masters in Human Nutrition and Functional Medicine. Dr. Hussey has worked with many people over the years and has seen the power of food, lifestyle change, and personal environment modification change lives every day. He coaches people across the world back to health at www.resourceyourhealth.com. When he is not working he enjoys time outdoors as well as reading, playing sports, and spending time with his wife and their three cats. *The Health Evolution* is Dr. Hussey's first book.

Index

E

F